Overweight

Withdrawn

Overweight

A Handbook for
Teens and Parents

Tania Heller, M.D.
Foreword by Mohsen Ziai, M.D.

McFarland & Company, Inc., Publishers
Jefferson, North Carolina, and London

LIBRARY OF CONGRESS CATALOGUING-IN-PUBLICATION DATA

Heller, Tania, 1958–
    Overweight: a handbook for teens and parents / Tania Heller ;
foreword by Mohsen Ziai.
       p.   cm.
    Includes bibliographical references and index.

    ISBN 0-7864-2082-0 (softcover : 50# alkaline paper)

    1. Obesity in adolescence — Popular works. 2. Obesity in
children — Popular works. I. Title.
RJ399.C6H45   2005
618.92'398 — dc22   2005004360

British Library cataloguing data are available

Cover photograph: ©2005 Image Source

Manufactured in the United States of America

McFarland & Company, Inc., Publishers
  Box 611, Jefferson, North Carolina 28640
  www.mcfarlandpub.com

A Message to the Readers

I wrote this book primarily for older teenagers and parents. Although it is equally important for children and younger teenagers to maintain a healthy lifestyle, I believe that their parents should guide them towards healthy eating patterns and being more active. Young children should learn the importance of good nutrition and physical activity for health and fitness, but I don't think that it is appropriate for them to delve into the intricacies of calories and food labels.

As a teenager, however, you will constantly be faced with decisions relating to eating and activity, and I am hopeful that the information in this book will guide you well. This is not a book about dieting — instead, it is about getting you started on a healthy path that you can maintain for the rest of your life.

Acknowledgments

I am so grateful to a large number of people who gave me advice and support while I was writing this book.

Thank you to Pamela Kanda, M.P.H., at the American Academy of Pediatrics, and to Kathy Toepfer, registered dietitian, for reviewing the section on nutrition and treatment.

I am grateful to psychiatrist Dr. E. James Lieberman and to my colleagues at the Suburban Center for Eating Disorders and Adolescent Obesity for everything they have taught me.

Thank you to Jackie Rommel for her dedication and support.

I also appreciate the help of the staffs of Walter Johnson and Walt Whitman high schools for their help with the lifestyle study and questionnaires.

Finally, a special thank you to my family for making me believe that anything worthy is possible, and to the young people who shared their stories with me. (Names and identifying characteristics have been changed to maintain confidentiality.)

Contents

Contents

Foreword

I have known Dr. Tania Heller for over two decades, first when she was a resident at Georgetown University Medical Center and rotated through our department at Fairfax Hospital, and later as a close friend. I have witnessed her numerous contributions to medical care as a pediatrician, teacher, radio host and author — some of the many ways she has given clear messages about a healthy way of life.

In this volume Dr. Heller has depicted the threat of obesity which, along with cigarette smoking, is a great danger to healthy living and yet is also preventable. Aside from predisposing the individual to life-threatening conditions such as diabetes, heart disease and iron deficiency, obesity is also a serious social issue associated with job discrimination, bullying in school and other psychological conditions.

Malnutrition and iron deficiency often coexist and are the world's number one causes of poor health. Malnutrition does not only refer to insufficient nutrition. It also includes over-consumption of the wrong nutrients: too much fat and carbohydrates instead of healthier foods (such as vegetables) and excessive intake of high-sugar sodas and juices instead of fresh fruits that provide better nutrition.

Dr. Heller has discussed some very important aspects of unhealthy nutrition and has presented several insightful case histories. You will read about the causes of obesity, its complications and associated problems, and how to get help. You will learn tips on healthy nutrition and physical activity. Instead of rushing to consume your food, or eating your sandwich while driving or using the cell phone, savor its taste. Eat nutritious foods including fruits and vegetables, and substitute taking a walk and even stopping to smell the flowers for at least some of the hours that you would spend watching television or sitting at the computer. Try to eat with the family around the table, and talk about the day's events. By making small changes now, you may prevent serious consequences later.

Both teenagers and their parents can learn much from this highly informative book.

Mohsen Ziai, M.D.

Chairman Emeritus, Department of Pediatrics,
Inova Fairfax Hospital for Children

Clinical Professor of Pediatrics,
University of Virginia School of Medicine

Professor Emeritus of Pediatrics,
University of Rochester School of Medicine

Lecturer in Pediatrics,
The Johns Hopkins University School of Medicine

Preface

More than twenty years ago, when I was treating malnourished patients in South Africa, I didn't imagine that one day one of our biggest healthcare crises would be related to excess food rather than insufficient food. Even poor children in the United States are more often affected by the problems related to being overweight than by hunger. Today it is evident that obesity among children and teenagers has reached epidemic proportions.

The lifestyles of most young Americans have changed dramatically with respect to physical activity as well as nutrition. Decades ago young people often walked for miles daily: to go to school, go shopping, visit their friends, or even see their doctor. There was no television to watch for hours on end, and instead of spending time chatting to friends on the Internet, they would have to make a quick phone call, or walk to pay them a visit. They played pick-up ball games instead of video games. In this regard, we must come to terms with the fact that our way of life may not be as healthy as it once was.

With respect to nutrition, there were few options when it came to snacks and cereals, and people rarely bought precooked meals or ate out at restaurants. Instead, families cooked at home, and spent time enjoying meals together. Today, with our advanced technology, foods have become more processed and abundant, and more choices are available. They are also tempting and cheap. Our lifestyles have become hurried, and we have become more accustomed to fast foods, which are usually less nutritious and and higher in sugars, carbohydrates and fats. Also, for some people, foods are used to fill a different kind of hunger — the emptiness and loneliness felt in today's fast-paced modern world.

All of these things have contributed to the rise in obesity, now being identified in younger and younger people. With the increase in childhood and adolescent obesity comes a high price — an increase in illnesses such as diabetes mellitus, high blood pressure, high cholesterol and even cancer. Also, overweight people usually suffer from low self-esteem, and may even become socially isolated, or develop depression or anxiety. Sadly, there is still prejudice related to obese people in our culture. This is evident by the fact that overweight people are more often rated negatively on their job performance. They are also less likely to find good jobs, or even social opportunities, than their thinner counterparts.

This may be the unfair reality, but it doesn't mean that you can't do something to change the situation. If you are overweight or not physically fit, you can make changes in your own lifestyle in order to become healthier and lose weight. You can also be an advocate and help promote changes in our society.

This book differs from many of the others on obesity, because it is aimed at young people like yourselves and your families. We cannot wait for a bigger crisis to occur (such as more people with diabetes and high blood pressure) before doing something about this problem. My goal in writing this book is to reach you before you develop the serious health problems and are confronted with social consequences too often seen in overweight people.

Now what may appear to be a paradox: I want to caution you against restrictive dieting. This can lead to serious problems including eating disorders, and can sometimes even lead to further weight gain over the long term. Cutting down drastically on calories can lead to a slower metabolism — making future weight loss much more difficult — or can lead to excessive hunger and bingeing. The best long-term way to maintain a healthy weight or prevent becoming overweight is a balanced eating plan — one of moderation, with healthy amounts of physical activity. We know diets hardly ever work, and people usually regain the weight they lost and more, so why does it seem that everyone is going on one diet after another? In a society accustomed to instant gratification, it's tempting to look for a quick fix or a magic answer. It may seem like too much effort to do what we know makes sense but takes so much time. After speaking to so many young people, however, I'm convinced that doing it the right way really does pay off in the end. There is no magic answer.

I wrote this book to help you determine whether you have a problem, and if you do, to help you find a solution. You will learn about why people become overweight as well as the problems that come from being overweight. I will also try to answer your questions, clear up some common misconceptions about weight and nutrition, and provide you with many resources for futher information. I am optimistic that it can help you get started on the right path. Through better lifestyle habits, good nutrition and increased physical activity, you will be on your way to becoming healthier and feeling better.

1

What Is Obesity?

Obesity is a serious chronic disease, defined by having too much body fat in relation to lean body mass. When referring to young people, the words obesity and overweight are often used interchangeably, and I will do so in this book.

Although overweight and obesity are quite clearly defined in adults, they are not as well defined in children and adolescents. A measure that is frequently used is the body mass index (BMI), a weight-for-height formula which corresponds well to total body fat. BMI is defined as weight in kilograms divided by height in meters squared (kg/m2). Another easy way to calculate your BMI is the following: Your body weight in pounds multiplied by 703, divided by your height in inches, squared. If you are 5 feet tall (60 inches) and weigh 100 pounds, you would multiply 100 by 703, then divide the product by 60, and then divide that by 60 again. Because normal body mass index changes with age in children and teenagers, and the guidelines are not the same as they are in adults, it's best to have your doctor interpret your body mass index and decide whether or not you are overweight and need treatment.

Your doctor can check your body mass index, and plot it on a standard BMI chart similar to the ones below to determine your risk. Obesity or overweight in children and teenagers is defined as a body mass index at or above the 95th percentile for age and sex. A BMI between the 85th and 95th percentiles means that one is at risk for obesity.

Remember that body mass index is only a guide, and should be looked at together with overall health. Although body mass index is a pretty reliable way to tell whether you are overweight, it doesn't take into account how muscular you are. If you are very muscular, your BMI may be high even though you don't have too much body fat.

Body Mass Index Chart: Girls 2–20 Years Old

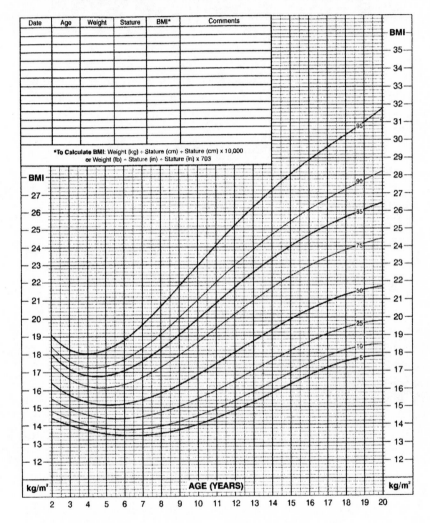

cdc/nchs

8

Body Mass Index Chart: Boys 2–20 Years Old

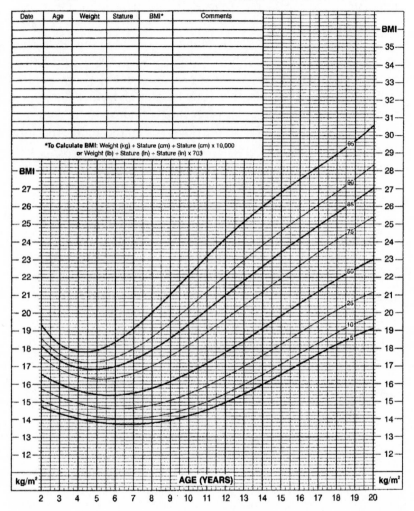

Date	Age	Weight	Stature	BMI*	Comments

*To Calculate BMI: Weight (kg) ÷ Stature (cm) ÷ Stature (cm) x 10,000
or Weight (lb) ÷ Stature (in) ÷ Stature (in) x 703

cdc/nchs

Copies of the standard body mass index charts for boys and girls are available from the National Center for Health Statistics; go to: www.cdc.gov/growthcharts.

Overweight

Approximately 15 percent of children and teenagers in the United States are considered overweight and many more are at risk. This number tripled from 1980 to 2000. The prevalence of young people who are overweight varies among different ethnic and racial groups: for example, the numbers are highest for Hispanic and Native American children and for African-American girls (CDC 1997; Crawford 2001; Ogden 1997). In the United States and other developed countries, being overweight also seems to be more common among poorer families. People living in poverty eat the foods that are cheaper, easier to get hold of, and which provide quick energy. These foods, which are often higher in sugars and fat, are more accessible than fresh fruits and vegetables. Obesity does not affect only the United States. It is a global problem. More and more children in Europe, the Middle East, Asia, South Africa, and other parts of the world are affected.

More than 60 percent of adults in the United States are either overweight or obese, and overweight children and teenagers are at high risk for becoming overweight adults. This is such a serious problem that its harmful effects have been compared to, and may soon even exceed, those of smoking. Sadly also, if we don't do something soon, today's generation of children may be the first generation that will have a shorter life-span than that of their parents' generation.

2

Why Do People Become Overweight, and Why Are So Many More Young People Overweight?

People gain weight when they take in more energy (food) than they use up. Do you know that eating or drinking 3500 extra calories will lead to a one-pound weight gain, so if you added one extra 16-ounce soda a day (200 calories), you could gain as many as 20 pounds over a year? People lose weight by expending more calories than they take in. So, by increasing your physical activity by only 50 calories per day, e.g. walking a half-mile, you could lose five pounds per year.

Many factors can cause or contribute to obesity. Although genetics plays an important role in determining whether someone is more likely to become overweight, the environment and lifestyle factors make it happen. The dramatic increase in the number of people with obesity over the last 20 years is related to changes in our environment, and not genetics. Twenty years is too short a time period for our gene pool to have changed that much.

Although it may seem obvious, people are still looking for a more specific answer to explain why so many young people are overweight in the 21st century. Many factors are being blamed for causing Americans to gain weight. Some people want to sue fast-food companies for misleading the American consumer. Many wonder whether restaurant owners are to blame for serving portions that are too large. Some are blaming schools for cutting physical education programs. Unfortunately, there is no one simple answer. It is a combination of things related to our changing environment that has led to the epidemic of obesity in the 21st century.

It may interest you to know that in the 1970s, during a time of relative scarcity, Americans demanded cheaper food. The government responded with policies that created huge surpluses and cheap foods. Snack foods were tempting and plentiful and portions became larger. What do you think we did? We responded by eating more. Believe it or not, today it is often cheaper to buy a ready-made (fast-food) dinner for an entire family than it is to cook one. Also, you can often pay less for a box of cookies or donuts than for a salad or even a piece of fruit.

Our environment is not what it was a few decades ago. Instead of pointing a finger, we must all take responsibility as soon as possible, accept the challenge, and discover ways to become a healthier society.

Weight gain can be caused by lifestyle factors such as poor nutrition and inactivity, genetics, medical conditions, binge-eating disorder, stress or depression, and medications. Now let's look at some of the causes in more detail.

Lifestyle Behaviors

Obesity is caused by an energy imbalance over a long period of time — in other words, by eating and drinking too many calories, and not getting enough physical activity. Our Westernized environment, with its abundant fast, cheap food, and energy-saving devices (e.g. elevators, escalators, remotes and cell phones), makes it easier for us to eat more, exercise less, and gain weight. As they adopt some of our behaviors, residents of other countries are following the trend. For example, as Italians adopt our fast-food culture and become more sedentary, they are seeing a sharp rise in the number of children and teenagers with obesity. This indicates to us how important lifestyle behaviors are when it comes to weight control.

Poor nutrition: Fast food, junk food, too much food

These days it takes more than just willpower and personal responsibility to maintain a healthy weight, so don't be too hard on yourself if you have struggled until now. The content of food as well as its availability is very different from what it was twenty years ago. Foods are more processed and often higher in calories, sugars and fats. Labels may be misleading because of portion size, etc. Foods are also more accessible at any time of day, almost anywhere, and can be eaten on the run. If you become hungry while driving home from school, you are sure to find a convenience store or a drive-through restaurant. In many hotels you can order room service around the clock, and in schools and even in hospitals, you will find vending machines or fast-food outlets.

Today, families eat more meals outside the home. They also eat more fast foods. The number of fast-food restaurants almost doubled from 1972 to 1995. This is important because a study found that children who ate fast foods took in more calories, fats and added sugars, and fewer fruits and non-starchy vegetables, than did those who ate no fast foods. Fast foods are often served in large portions, are usually low in fiber, and appeal to the tastes of many people. I asked a student why he ate at one of the fast-food restaurants so often, and he replied: "Because you get a good deal." People also eat at fast-food restaurants because it's convenient and it's quick. Because of their busy lifestyles, many people don't have time to prepare food at home. Eating out also means they won't have to clean up and wash dishes. Running in to buy a burger, fries and a Coke may seem like the perfect solution to them. Poor people may have better access to these and other high-calorie, high-fat foods, and less access to fresh fruits and vegetables. Also, fast foods sometimes cost less than more nutritious foods. Unfortunately, much of the marketing is directed at very young children, who are not in a position to make the best health choices for themselves. They are lured in not only by the food, but also by the toys, the clowns and the playgrounds. Once they become "hooked," it's hard to break their fast-food habit. All of these factors may promote a greater intake of fast foods, which in turn can contribute to obesity.

Another factor I believe contributes to the obesity crisis is that families don't sit down to meals together on a regular basis. Instead of eating balanced home-cooked meals, they often eat on the run, buy ready-made food, or skip meals and replace them with snacks. All of these habits can result in taking in less of the nutritious foods like fruits, vegetables and dairy products, and more "empty" calories.

We are also snacking more. Never before has there been such a variety of snack foods. There are snacks for every occasion and for every time of day. Everywhere we see ads for the latest snack food — on billboards, on television, and in magazines. The problem with this is that the more high-calorie, high-carbohydrate and high-fat foods are available to us, the more we will eat. It was found that in general, when people are given larger portions, they will eat more, rather than regulate themselves. Many people say that the amount of food they eat depends on how much food they are served rather than how hungry they are. Portions have become much larger in restaurants, and now also at home. Restaurants attract customers by offering giant-sized burgers or sandwiches and extra-large sodas. Buffet ads promise all-you-can-eat meals. For many it may seem difficult or even wasteful to pass up these offers. Remember being taught to "clean your plate"?

Also, young people are exposed to vending machines with candies and sodas, not only on the streets and in shopping malls, but even in hospitals and in schools. Many schools depend on food and beverage companies to supplement their funding, and the highest bidder wins. In addition to vending machines, schools may have snack bars or stores, or bake sales and other fundraisers with students selling candy or cookies. Moreover, clever marketing entices us to buy more. For example, mini-sized chocolates come in large "extra-value" bags. Instead of buying one regular-sized bar of chocolate, you may buy the bag of mini chocolates, thinking that you are saving money, and that the chocolates are smaller. However, because you have a large bag of chocolates, you are more likely to eat more than you would have if you had simply bought one regular chocolate bar.

2. Why Do People Become Overweight

Some people may buy foods because they imagine them to be more nutritious than they are. Nutrition information on food packaging is not always accurate. Terms such as "light," "natural" or low-fat can be misleading.

Teenagers also drink a large number of fruit juices and soft drinks, which may add hundreds of calories and take the place of healthier drinks such as water and milk. It appears as though calories in the form of liquids (soft drinks) may not be perceived by the body as well as calories in the form of solid foods. In other words, you can take in more than you realize without feeling full, and may not compensate by eating fewer calories later. This was not as much of an issue in the past, but with serving sizes up to three times as large as they were in the 1950s, this can have a big impact on health. Besides adding extra calories, drinking sweetened drinks can lead to dental caries and calcium deficiency, because of displacement of milk in the diet. Soft drink intake has increased by 300 percent in twenty years. More than half of schoolchildren drink at least one soft drink every day, with some drinking four or more servings a day.

On the other hand, while young people are eating more calories, fewer than 15 percent of schoolchildren get the recommended number of servings of fruits and vegetables a day. When they do eat vegetables, they're not always the best type. Would you believe that a quarter of all vegetables eaten in the United States are French fries? As you can see, the environment is not very supportive of people who do want to be healthier, but this doesn't mean you have to give up. There are things you can do to counteract this. I have seen some positive changes even while writing this book. Schools are now starting to provide healthier options in vending machines, and restaurant chains are making nutritional information available to their customers. School lunch programs still need to be improved. I testified in Annapolis, the capital of my home state of Maryland, in favor of a bill to improve the lunch programs. There's a lot that still needs to be done before we can relax.

Below I have listed some of the poor eating habits I see in many teenagers. See if you recognize any of these habits in yourself:

- Skipping breakfast
- Snacking all day
- Eating too many fast foods
- Mindless eating while doing other things
- Restrictive eating/skipping meals and binge eating
- Too few fruits and vegetables
- Too little calcium
- Too many sodas and snacks high in sugars and fat
- Yo-yo dieting
- Eating late at night
- Eating for reasons other than hunger, e.g. when bored

If you do identify with any of these, normalizing your eating patterns needs to be one of your first goals—even before weight loss.

Inactivity

One of the biggest culprits in our weight crisis is that young people are not as active as they once were. In fact, children tend to become less active as they progress through the teenage years. Because they are eating at least as much as, if not more than, young people used to eat in the past, and not burning it off with physical activity, they are gaining weight. Although many teenagers in the United States are active and participate in sports, many are still too sedentary. I have heard from many young people (and adults) that they watch well over four hours of television daily, and many also spend a significant amount of time playing video games or sitting at the computer.

Here are some of the reasons that young people may not be as active as they should be:

- Safety concerns: Because of safety concerns, parents may be less willing to let their children play or bike outdoors. Many families also live in areas with poor access to parks and sidewalks. When we were kids and off from school we played outside until dark. Today children are more likely to sit inside and watch television.
- School physical education cuts: Many schools, especially those with

poor financial resources, have done away with mandatory physical education programs to make time and funding available for other "more important" programs. If you are a student this may have a negative impact on your health, especially if you don't participate in much physical activity outside of school.

- Sitting on the sidelines: Teenagers have told me that students who are not very athletic don't get picked for teams and don't get called to play often. It's sad, because these may be the students who could benefit most from the physical activity.
- Time constraints: Families today are very busy. Often both parents are working and this makes it difficult to arrange activities together — activities such as a family walk or hike, or bike riding together. I asked a mother of a young boy what her son did for exercise. She said that she didn't really know whether he was active during the day, as she didn't see him until 7 P.M. when she came home from work. And as we know, this has unfortunately become the norm for many working families. You yourself may identify with this if both your parents work outside the home.
- Poverty: Children living in poverty may have less access to parks and playgrounds.
- Television: In a 1998 Nielson Media research report on television viewing, it was revealed that the average American child or teenager spends more than twenty-one hours a week watching TV — that's three hours a day! This did not take into account other media and computer time. More time involved in these sedentary activities leaves less time for physical activity. Also, watching television exposes you to constant snack-food commercials, and food commercials that are broadcast during children's and teens' programming often promote high-calorie foods. In fact, more than 60 percent of television commercials during children's programs are food-related. Not only are you encouraged to eat these foods, but you may be less aware of how much you eat while watching television. Studies show that watching more than two hours of television a day significantly increases your likelihood of becoming overweight. How much television do you watch each day?
- Other sedentary behaviors: Apart from watching television, many

young people spend several hours a day sitting in front of their computers, watching movies or playing video games.

Where you live

A study found that people who live in neighborhoods in which they can easily walk to their destinations—such as the local store or pharmacy—are less likely to be obese. In fact, for every kilometer (half-mile) they walked in a day, they were 5 percent less likely to be obese (*Time* magazine, June 7, 2004). Those who depend on their cars to go everywhere have a tendency to gain weight. Some suburban neighborhoods lack sidewalks and don't have shops that are easily accessible by foot. People living there walk less and are at risk for weight gain.

Genetics

Genes play a big role in determining whether someone will become overweight, but the genetics of obesity is complicated and a large number of genes are probably involved. Obesity runs in families. Young children with parents of normal weight have only a small chance of developing severe weight problems. However, if one parent is obese, the odds ratio for obesity in adulthood increases to about 3, and if both parents are obese, the ratio further increases to more than 10. If you are already overweight and you have at least one overweight parent, you have a much higher chance of being overweight when you are an adult (Donohoue 2004; Amer. Acad. of Pediatrics, Committee on Nutrition, August 2003). Most likely, this is caused by both genetic and environmental factors. You may inherit your parents' genes, but you may also mimic their eating and other lifestyle behaviors. Don't be discouraged, though. Although there is not much you can do to change your genetic make-up, there is a whole lot you can do to change your lifestyle habits, and so lessen your chances of becoming overweight.

A great amount of research is being done to determine which genes are associated with obesity and involved in determining hunger and satiety. Although there have been many discoveries in the last few years, we still don't have all the answers to our questions. If you look at genetic causes of obesity, most people become overweight due to the effect of multiple genes. However, there are some specific genetic conditions and syndromes caused by defects in single genes, and I have listed some of these below.

Some Medical Conditions Associated with Obesity

A variety of genetic, hormonal, and other problems have obesity as one of their indicators.

Genetic problems and syndromes

Although genetics (the genes you inherit from your parents) plays a big role in determining weight, genetic syndromes account for less than 1 percent of childhood obesity. Most people become overweight because of lifestyle behaviors or because one or both of their parents are overweight. Children with genetic syndromes are usually short, whereas those who become overweight due to lifestyle behaviors are usually tall.

- Prader-Willi syndrome: This is a genetic disorder associated with low muscle tone in infancy, ravenous appetite, childhood obesity, short stature, and mental deficiency.
- Bardet-Biedl syndrome: This autosomal-recessive, genetic syndrome is also associated with obesity, short stature and mental retardation. Also, patients with this disorder may have numerous other problems, such as hearing loss, loss of sight, kidney abnormalities and speech problems.
- Alstrom syndrome: This is a rare autosomal-recessive genetic disorder. Affected patients have early-onset obesity, visual and hearing impairment, heart problems and diabetes.
- Cohen syndrome: This is another rare genetic disorder associated with obesity, severe mental retardation and short stature.
- Down syndrome: This syndrome is caused by a chromosomal abnormality and is associated with hypotonia (low muscle tone) and obesity.

- Leptin deficiency: Deficiency of the hormone leptin, which is produced primarily by fat cells, is a rare cause of excessive hunger and obesity.
- Other genetic problems: A defect (mutation) in the melanocortin 4 (MC4) receptor gene was found in a study to be associated with binge eating.

Hormonal problems

Hormonal problems such as hypothyroidism and Cushing syndrome (hypercortisolism) are rare causes of obesity. A thorough history and physical examination will usually give clues to these diagnoses. Individuals with hypothyroidism gain some weight, and may complain of symptoms such as constipation and feeling cold all the time. Lab tests will reveal low thyroid hormone (T4) levels and an elevated TSH (thyroid-stimulating hormone) level. Patients with Cushing syndrome have central (trunk) obesity and slowing of their growth in height. To make the diagnosis, tests are done to demonstrate high cortisol levels. There are other hormonal conditions, such as elevated insulin levels (primary hyperinsulinism) or conditions involving the hypothalamus (tumors, infection or trauma), that can also lead to obesity. These are rare. Medical scientists are studying additional hormones and neurotransmitters that appear to be involved in regulating hunger. These include growth hormone, ghrelin, neuropeptide Y and others.

Other medical conditions

Polycystic ovary syndrome (Stein-Leventhal syndrome), in which individuals have multiple cysts on the ovaries, leads to irregular menstrual cycles, excess unwanted hair on the body or face, and being overweight. Many women with polycystic ovary syndrome (PCOS) have insulin resistance or diabetes, and the syndrome can also be a cause of infertility. Some patients may develop acne, have mood swings, or even depression. The exact cause of polycystic ovary syndrome is still unknown, but studies are being done to look at a possible genetic cause and to look at its relation to insulin production (because of its association with diabetes). If you think you may have symptoms of PCOS, speak to your primary-care doctor who will assess you for the disorder, and help you with treatment options if necessary. Treatment may include medication, and weight loss if the person is overweight.

Interaction Between Genes and the Environment

A long time ago when humans had to obtain food through strenuous physical activity such as hunting, and they were faced with the constant threat of hunger and famine, genotypes developed to favor energy storage. These are known as "thrifty" genes. They operate as though they don't know when you will have your next meal — as though you were a hunter in the field. Today, in our environment of plentiful, readily available, high-calorie food, these "thrifty" genotypes have become harmful and promote weight gain and the storage of fat. This is an example of how genetics and our environment have interacted together to increase the prevalence of obesity.

Binge–Eating Disorder

Some people who are overweight have an eating disorder — binge-eating disorder. This is an illness in which individuals (male or female) have recurrent episodes of binge eating, in which they eat large amounts of food in an out-of-control manner, and often have feelings of guilt or shame after the binge. Binge-eating disorder is the most common eating disorder and can occur along with both medical and psychiatric conditions. It usually begins in the late teens or early twenties, but people sometimes present for treatment much later.

Negative childhood experiences and a tendency to become overweight can put one at risk for developing binge-eating disorder, as can low self-esteem and living in a culture that emphasizes thinness. Severe calorie restrictions can cause excessive hunger and cravings, and binge eating. People with binge-eating disorder often have several failed attempts at losing weight, and are often, but not always, overweight. [A later chapter discusses binge-eating disorder in more detail.]

Night Eating Syndrome

Dr. Albert Stunkard and his colleagues first identified a problem known as night eating syndrome in which patients eat most of their daily calories in the evening and at night, have a lack of appetite in the morning, and have difficulties with sleep. They may also have symptoms of depression. Because of their overeating in the later part of the day, they may be, but are not always, overweight.

Stress and Depression

Loneliness, family, or school problems may cause some people to overeat and gain weight. There are people who turn to food during stressful times, rather than dealing with their feelings. Also, individuals who suffer from depression may have changes in their eating patterns. Some lose appetite and may lose weight, and others eat excessively and gain weight.

Medications

Certain medications, such as steroids, and some antidepressants, are associated with weight gain.

Mixed Messages from Our Society

There is no question that our society gives us mixed messages. While sending a loud and clear message that thin and muscular are beautiful and that teenagers should diet to lose weight and spend lots of money on fitness products, our society is also promoting overeating by super-sizing, and by making high-calorie foods available everywhere. This can be very confusing to people, many of whom end up as chronic dieters.

There are even more challenges you may have to deal with in your efforts to remain at a healthy weight. Foods that are not as healthy for you taste good. Let's be honest—chocolate cake and ice cream are tempting. You are also likely to be exposed to a large number of food commercials or ads on television or in magazines, some of which give misleading information. Moreover, if you are like most teenagers, you are probably very busy, and may not always find the time to sit down to a home-cooked meal. This means that you may eat on the run, and eat fast foods more often.

I spoke to a student from Belgium who had been studying in the United States for a few years. I asked him what differences he had noticed in lifestyle behaviors between Belgian and American students. He didn't hesitate for a moment. "Everyone is so hurried here. They can't relax. There is so much pressure to do well at school and at work. There is even pressure placed on sports and activities that should be fun. American students are too stressed." I asked about the food in Belgium, and he told me: "I haven't had a good slice of bread since I left. At home we also used to sit down with the family for proper meals rather than eating so much fast food. That allowed us to be able to eat an occasional Belgian chocolate. I miss having relaxing meals. We don't make time to do that here."

What You Can Control

Although there are a number of causes of obesity, the causes that you can influence most easily are lifestyle factors and your behaviors.

Questionnaire on lifestyle habits

I did a study at two local schools, asking 9th and 10th grade students to fill out the following questionnaire about their lifestyle habits. A summary of their responses follows the questionnaire. Feel free to fill it out yourself and see how your lifestyle habits compare to theirs.

Where appropriate, check the most accurate response to each question.

1. What is your age? _____ years.
2. Are you male ? _____ female ? _____

3. How often do you eat breakfast in the morning?
   Every morning _____
   4–6 mornings a week _____
   Fewer than 4 mornings a week _____
4. Do you pack a lunch to take to school? _____
   Do you buy/receive lunch at school? _____
5. How often do you eat take-out and/or eat at restaurants?
   Fewer than 3 times a week _____
   3–4 times a week _____
   More than 4 times a week _____
6. Approximately how many regular (non-diet) sodas do you drink every week?
   7 or more _____
   2–6 _____
   Fewer than 2 _____
7. How often do you drink fruit juice?
   Daily _____
   Often _____
   Sometimes _____
   Almost never _____
8. How many servings of fruits and vegetables do you get every day?
   5 or more _____
   4 _____
   Fewer than 4 _____
9. How many servings of milk, cheese or yogurt do you eat or drink each day?
   At least 3 servings _____
   1–2 servings _____
   Fewer than 1 serving _____
10. How often do you use a vending machine to buy food or drink?
   4 or more days a week _____
   1–3 days a week _____
   Never _____
11. On average, weekdays and weekends, how many hours of television do you watch?
   More than 4 hours a day _____

3–4 hours a day _____

1½–3 hours a day _____

Fewer than 1½ hours a day _____

12. Do you have a television set in your bedroom?

Yes _____

No _____

13. How often do you eat while you watch television?

A lot _____

Sometimes _____

Never _____

14. How much time do you spend at the computer (including homework) and playing video games (combined)?

2 or more hours a day _____

1–2 hours a day _____

Less than 1 hour a day _____

15. Do you participate in school physical education (P.E.)?

Yes _____

No _____

16. Apart from school P.E., how often do you exercise for 30 minutes or more?

Every day _____

4–6 days a week _____

Fewer than 4 days a week _____

Over one hundred questionnaires were randomly handed out to ninth and tenth graders in two different East Coast high schools. Sixty-six responded by completing the questionnaire — 27 males and 39 females. The following is a summary of their responses.

Only 30 of the 66 students said they eat breakfast every morning, and 23 (about 35 percent) reported that they eat breakfast fewer than four mornings a week. Thirty-five buy or receive lunch at school. Fourteen eat out or order take-out at least three times a week. Nineteen drink at least two regular sodas a week and only five reported that they drink more than seven regular sodas per week. Twenty-six drink fruit juice daily. Only 13 (about 20 percent) said they get the recommended five or more servings of fruits and vegetables a day, while 26 (almost 40 percent) get fewer than four servings. Twenty-seven students (less than half) said they get at least three servings of milk products daily.

When it came to the use of vending machines to buy food or drinks, about half (30) said they never use a vending machine, while the other half (31) said they use a vending machine one to three days a week. Fifteen students (about 23 percent) said that they watch television for at least three hours a day. As many as 21 students (about a third) have television sets in their bedrooms. Apart from watching television, 30 students (almost half) said they spend two or more hours a day at the computer and/or playing video games. Twenty eat a lot while watching television. Only 35 students (53 percent) said they participate in school physical education and 48 exercise for a half-hour (outside of school P.E.) on four to six days a week. Twelve students did not participate in P.E. and exercised fewer than 4 days a week.

How do you compare to them?

Are you at risk for obesity or excessive weight gain?

Take this informal test:

1. Is one (or are both) of your parents overweight?
2. Do you watch television for 1½ hours or more a day?
3. Do you eat out or order take-out more than twice a week?
4. Do you regularly engage in binge eating, i.e. eating very large amounts of food in a short period of time, in an out-of-control manner?
5. Do you drink sodas or juice on most days?
6. Do you eat fewer than four servings of fruits and vegetables daily?
7. Do you participate in physical activity (half-hour or more) less than four days per week?

If you answered yes to two or more of the above, you may be at increased risk for obesity or further excessive weight gain.

3

Binge-Eating Disorder

While consuming too many calories and getting too little exercise is by far the most common cause of obesity; some overweight people do suffer from an eating disorder: binge-eating disorder.

Barry's Story

Barry, now adult, spoke openly for the first time about his bingeing. "I have lived with this problem for years and have never felt comfortable speaking about it. For a long time I thought I was the only one suffering from something like this. My eating problem has affected every aspect of my life. I spend most of my days thinking about food. I think about food when I wake up in the morning and when I go to bed at night. I also think about food at work and keep stacks of candy in my desk drawer. It has affected my relationships, my social life and my work. Often I arrive home late because I stop at a restaurant or a drug store, and I've even left important meetings to go to the vending machine for snacks."

I asked Barry whether there was anything that triggered his binges. "Situations, such as parties, buffets and other functions, certain people, and most of all, if I had a stressful day," he said. "The binge lifts my mood only temporarily, and then I feel so much worse. It's a vicious cycle." I asked Barry if he exercised at all and whether he felt that exercising made a difference. "On the days I exercise, I binge less. I don't seem to have as enormous an appetite after exercising, and it also improves my mindset. I feel better about myself when I'm active, so I binge less." "What else helps?" I asked. "Structure is key. When I stick to my standard routine and have planned meals, and exercise, I do so much better."

What is Binge-Eating Disorder?

Binge-eating disorder (BED) is the most common known eating disorder. Individuals with BED have recurrent binge eating, but unlike people with bulimia, they don't have regular episodes of purging, excessive exercising, or severe restriction. Most, but not all, patients are overweight. Symptoms of binge-eating disorder include:

. Regular episodes of eating unusually large quantities of food in relatively short periods of time. During a binge, they often eat even when not hungry, eat much more quickly than usual, and eat until they are uncomfortable.
. A sense of lack of control over the eating behavior.
. Distress over their eating behavior.
. The binges occur at least two days a week for six months.

Remember that if you occasionally overeat, it does not mean that you have binge-eating disorder!

Who Develops BED?

About 3 percent of adults in the community suffer from binge-eating disorder, but as many as 15 to 30 percent of patients seeking treatment for obesity are found to have the illness. Females are affected slightly more often than males: about 60 percent are female. People most often present for treatment only after the age of thirty, although I have had many teenagers tell me that they engage in binge eating. Most but not all people with binge-eating disorder are overweight.

Complications of Binge-Eating Disorder

These are similar to the complications seen with obesity, and include high blood pressure, high blood cholesterol, heart and gallbladder disease and Type 2 diabetes. People with binge-eating disorder may also become depressed. Their illness can cause them a lot of distress, and this can lead them to become socially isolated. Some people spend large amounts of money on food for binges. One teenager told me that she once drove to three different grocery stores to buy food for a binge, because she was too embarrassed to buy all that food at one time.

What Causes BED?

The cause of binge-eating disorder is not known, but there are several contributing factors. People who have a tendency towards being overweight, or who have been exposed to teasing or negative comments about their weight, are at risk for binge eating. Researchers have discovered a link between a defect in a receptor on a gene (the melanocortin 4 receptor) and binge eating. There is also an association between depression and binge eating, although it is unknown whether depression is a cause or an effect. It does seem as if people with binge-eating disorder have an increased likelihood of having parents or other family members with depression. Binges may be triggered by a variety of events. Severe calorie restriction can trigger binge eating. Binges can also be triggered by all sorts of emotions, including being sad, stressed or bored.

Treatment

Treatment of binge-eating disorder usually involves some form of psychotherapy, with or without medication. If you suffer from binge-eating disorder, work with your doctor or therapist to establish realistic goals for yourself. The first goals of treatment should be to decrease your bingeing, normalize your eating behavior, and improve your coping skills. You can then focus on weight loss, if necessary. If you think you may have binge-eating disorder, don't try to manage this on your own. Get help from a health professional. You can start with your primary-care physician, who may refer you to a different specialist if necessary. Remember that you are not alone, and treatment is available.

4

Interviews with Teenagers

Many overweight teenagers are dissatisfied with their bodies and suffer from low self-esteem. Some isolate themselves and don't socialize with friends, for fear that they may be rejected because of their size. Unfortunately, in our society, which places a high value on thinness, overweight people are often teased and victimized. This is not acceptable and people should become more educated about this issue.

There are ethnic differences in the way people view their own bodies and what they perceive as an ideal body. In general, African-American women seem to be less affected than Caucasian women by our society's emphasis on thinness. However, a study found that obese African-American women are still less satisfied with their bodies than are non-obese African-American women.

Lisa's Story

Lisa is a ninth-grader who was at a healthy weight until eighth grade, after which her weight silently crept up. She did not believe that her lifestyle was very different from that of her friends, so she was surprised when she gained the weight. The following is an example of what a typical school day for her used to be:

Lisa was awakened by her alarm at 6:30 A.M. She showered, dressed and had a hurried breakfast of sweetened cereal and apple juice. She was usually just in time for her ride to school at 7:15. Lunch was at 11 A.M. in the school cafeteria. Her parents had signed her up to receive prepared lunches at school so that she could save time in the mornings. Lunches varied from day to day, but were usually some form of pasta or pizza. Her favorite lunch was baked pasta with cheese sauce, salad, and juice. For dessert, Lisa bought either a bag of chips or a cookie in the cafeteria, and then returned to class. Lisa was a good student and enjoyed school on most days. The school day was long, however, because frequently she had to stay after school until 5:00 when her mother picked her up. By 4:00 she was ravenously hungry, and because she didn't usually pack a snack, she relied on the vending machine which carried only chips, pretzels, chocolate or cookies. Lisa missed lower school. For one thing, she used to leave school earlier. Also, she had really enjoyed her regular "phys. ed." classes. In ninth grade, P.E. was no longer mandatory and she felt she was not getting much physical activity at all.

By the time she returned home after school it was 5:30 P.M. and Lisa barely had time to finish her homework before dinner. On some nights the whole family would sit down to dinner together, but on the nights her parents worked late, it was up to Lisa and her older brother to fend for themselves. They would microwave leftovers, or order Chinese food or pizza to be delivered to the house. If she had no more homework to do, Lisa would then watch television until her parents returned from work. After chatting with her parents for a few minutes, it was computer time, and time to check in with friends. She developed the habit of snacking on cookies or popcorn while sitting at the computer.

On weekends, Lisa usually slept until 11:00, and would often skip breakfast, and snack more. She did take part in a dance class on Saturdays, but also spent much more time watching television on the weekends.

You could say that Lisa was a typical ninth-grader. At the end of ninth grade, however, she was twenty pounds overweight.

Mark's Story

Mark is a sixteen-year-old who struggled with his weight for years and began to make significant changes in his lifestyle habits about a year ago. He went about it in a healthy way, gradually increasing his physical activity, and cutting down on portion sizes, as well as sugars and fats. He has lost fifty-five pounds and feels fitter and healthier than ever before. I asked him how he felt about the changes he had made.

"I was very, very happy when I accomplished my goal. When I was thirteen, my doctor said I needed to lose weight. I tried many different diets, but they didn't work for me, partly because they left no room for flexibility, and I also felt that they placed too little emphasis on exercise. It was really hard for me to get motivated, and I was very unhappy with the results. Last summer, I watched a television program on the health benefits of exercise, and then read an interesting article on health and nutrition, which was really the turning point for me. The article inspired me to eat better and exercise more. On the first day, I ran a little, and felt tired but good. Over the summer, I continued doing some activity almost every day, such as walking, or sometimes going for a run. I began cutting back on sweets, and although it was hard at first, I kept feeling better and better. I asked my parents to help by buying healthier foods and grilling or baking dinners instead of frying them. I continued to lose weight, and started approaching my goal weight."

"So the thing that really motivated you was the article on health?" I asked Mark. "That, and to some extent my Dad, as I really want him to become healthier too." I asked Mark what keeps him motivated, and he told me that feeling healthier, as well as positive reinforcement from friends and family were strong motivators. "I have more energy and feel much better about myself. I am also more confident. People do treat me differently now. Of course I am the same person as I was, and friends always liked my personality, but they teased me about my weight, and I really didn't like that. I don't get teased now. I definitely think our society stigmatizes overweight people, and that's sad."

"What is the most difficult part of sticking to your new routine? I asked Mark. "Pushing myself to exercise sometimes. But I decide to just do it. It also helps to have a friend to work out with and to motivate me." When asked what he would recommend to others wanting to become fitter and healthier, he said: "I guess I'll have to say, stick with it and you'll succeed!"

Rick's Story

Rick is also sixteen and has lost twenty pounds by exercising more and making healthier food choices. He says that the biggest benefit has been that he feels healthier. He has more stamina and can enjoy sports activities much more than he did before. I asked him what motivated him to change his habits. "The fact that I knew I was overweight. I did it mostly for health reasons. A friend also motivated me. He had begun to make healthy changes and I saw that he had success. I knew I could do it too. The most difficult time was early on — making those first changes, but as time goes on, habits change, and it has become much easier and feels natural being more active, and eating more healthily. Also, because I feel so much better, it's worth keeping up." I asked Rick whether people treated him differently after his weight loss, but he had not really noticed a change, although he agreed that there was some prejudice in our society, so that some people were treated differently on the basis of their size.

"So, what would you recommend to other teenagers who want to follow your example?" I asked. "Start by making one small change at a time. When that becomes habit, make the next change. For example, you can start by cutting out French fries, then going for walks, then adding more sports. Pretty soon you'll develop new healthier habits that will stay with you."

Rachel's Story

Fifteen-year-old Rachel told me: "There is so much pressure from society to look a certain way and to be thin. We shouldn't be worrying so much about the way we look, but I think most people do. I would like to lose some weight, but I am not obsessed by it. I probably wouldn't worry about my weight so much if all my friends weren't dieting. My one friend is on and off "Slim-Fast" and I have another friend who developed anorexia and was almost hospitalized." I asked Rachel if she had ever dieted.

"I was on Weight Watchers last year and I lost nine pounds, but I gained the weight back. I can't stick to any diet! It's kind of tough at my school because the other girls in my grade are so thin. They don't really tease the overweight kids but I do hear them make comments about who is fat."

Rachel told me that while she has to struggle so much with her weight, she has a sister who can eat anything and remains skinny. "It's so frustrating. She is always baking or buying candy and leaving it around the house. I find it very hard to resist these temptations, so every time I pass a cake, I'll take another bite. With just a bite each time, I don't feel as if I'm eating much, but obviously it all adds up. I don't weigh myself, but I can tell by the way my clothes fit. I know my sister doesn't do it on purpose, because I don't think she really understands what I go through. She has her own struggles. But it definitely makes it more difficult when everyone eats differently and temptations are everywhere. I wish I could have more control."

Rachel and I spoke about her body image and self-esteem and I asked her how she felt about her body and about herself as a person. "I feel good about who I am. I am okay with the way I look although I would change some things if I could. Some days I spend a lot of time worrying about it and about my weight, but not every day. It depends a lot on who I'm with. Also, when I read some of those fashion magazines and see those models, I definitely feel worse about myself. It's hard to have to compare yourself to those skinny models. Would I prefer to be in the top ten in my grade or lose 10 pounds this year? Gosh, I don't know. It's hard to say."

Marie's Story

Marie is a fifteen-year-old African-American girl with sparkling eyes and a beautiful smile. She is intelligent and creative and has supportive family and friends. Marie is also one hundred pounds overweight. All her family members have struggled with weight problems and her father and aunt both had gastric-bypass surgery when everything else failed. Marie was reluctantly brought to a doctor who specialized in weight problems, but seemed resigned to the fact that she too would fail. "It's just so hard," she told me, with tears in her eyes. "You have no idea. Do you know what it's like aching when you get up in the morning, then having a hard time putting on your socks? Do you know what it's like going to school feeling disgusted with yourself and knowing everyone is looking at you? I feel guilty eating in front of people, and I feel like the odd one out in P.E. I always wonder if my friends talk to me only because they feel sorry for me. And then all the time I think — and this is never going to get better. It's no need exercising and dieting when I know I'll end up having surgery one day. Why can't I have the surgery now?"

Her physician explained that surgery was a last resort for young people and that even if she did eventually need surgery, any positive lifestyle changes and safe weight loss now would lessen her surgical risks later. He also explained that she would have to work on her emotions around eating and explore ways other than eating to cope with stress and feelings. These issues would not go away with surgery. Although Marie still found it difficult to commit to change, she began to understand that surgery wasn't a quick fix.

5

Why Is Being Overweight a Problem?

Obesity is a serious, chronic illness that can lead to long-term medical and psychological complications. If we don't do something about the obesity crisis now, the problem will only get worse. Being overweight as a child or teenager puts you at increased risk for being overweight as an adult. It also puts you at risk for all the obesity-related complications seen in adults. An overweight four-year-old has a 20 percent chance of becoming an obese adult. If you are overweight as a teenager, the likelihood increases to 80 percent! When someone is overweight, there is an increase in the number and size of their fat cells. The number of fat cells in the body increases rapidly during childhood and puberty, but may continue to increase even as an adult. When a person loses weight, most fat loss occurs as a result of a decrease in the *size* of fat cells. Although long-term significant fat loss may also decrease the *number* of fat cells, once fat cells are formed, their number remains relatively fixed, and it seems to be difficult to lose them. There is a lot we don't yet know about this process and much research is being done to increase our understanding. Below you will read about the medical and psychological complications found in adults who are overweight. Today we are recognizing many of these problems in younger people too.

Medical Complications of Obesity

Diabetes

Diabetes mellitus is a chronic metabolic illness in which patients have high blood glucose (sugar) levels, because the body either produces too little insulin, or is resistant to (not responding to) its insulin. Insulin is a hormone made by the pancreas, and its role is to move glucose out of the bloodstream into various cells in the body. When this process breaks down, blood glucose levels rise. A person with Type 1 diabetes has high glucose levels because the pancreas no longer makes insulin. Such a person will need to have insulin shots as part of treatment. On the other hand, someone with Type 2 diabetes has enough insulin, but the body doesn't respond to it adequately. This is known as insulin resistance, and is often seen in people who are overweight. Not everyone who has insulin resistance has full-blown diabetes already, but it is a wake-up call to do something. Being overweight, therefore, increases one's risk of developing insulin resistance, or diabetes, with its serious complications such as heart disease, stroke, kidney disease and blindness.

Type 2 diabetes in young people has increased dramatically in the past several years. The large increase in the number of young people with this disease seems to be directly related to the increase in the number of young people who are overweight. The good news is that Type 2 diabetes and insulin resistance are usually preventable with weight control and lifestyle adjustments.

Metabolic syndrome

Another condition that can put one at risk for diabetes and early heart disease is known as the metabolic syndrome. People who have this syndrome have some combination of the following symptoms: an elevated fasting glucose level or insulin resistance, high blood pressure, low levels of high-density lipoprotein (HDL) cholesterol (good cholesterol), high fasting triglyceride levels, and a large waist size. Metabolic syndrome is believed to affect nearly one million teenagers in the United States, and it is a preventable illness.

Heart disease

Heart problems can occur even in young people who are overweight. Carrying extra weight puts added strain on the heart, or at the very least, makes it more difficult to be physically active, or even perform day-to-day activities. Diabetes, high cholesterol levels, high blood pressure and being overweight can all increase your risk for developing heart disease.

High cholesterol

High blood cholesterol levels and lipid abnormalities can be related to diet and obesity. Cholesterol is a substance found in some foods but is also made by the liver. High cholesterol levels can therefore be a result of genetics, but can also be caused by eating too many foods high in saturated fats and cholesterol. One type of cholesterol known as low-density lipoprotein (LDL) or "bad cholesterol" increases deposits on artery walls, narrowing them. This can lead to a condition called atherosclerosis (in which arteries are blocked with plaque) and heart disease. On the other hand, high-density lipoprotein (HDL) or "good cholesterol" helps to clear the deposits, and can therefore help protect against heart disease. Ask your doctor to check your blood cholesterol levels if you are overweight, have diabetes or high blood pressure, or if you have a family history of high cholesterol or heart disease.

Hypertension

High blood pressure, also known as hypertension, is found more often in overweight children and teenagers. It occurs when the pressure of the blood as it is being pumped through the arteries is higher than normal. Hypertension is a serious condition because it can cause damage to many organ systems in the body and can increase one's risk of developing heart disease. By staying at a healthy weight you will be less likely to develop high blood pressure.

Respiratory problems

Carrying too much extra body weight can make all activities, even breathing, more difficult. People suffering from asthma may have worse symptoms if they are overweight. People who are overweight may snore, and those with severe obesity can develop a dangerous condition known as sleep apnea, in which people stop breathing for short periods of time while they are asleep. Children with sleep apnea can develop problems with learning and memory.

Orthopedic problems

Carrying extra body weight can put added stress on joints, including knees, ankles, hips and back. In young children, bones may not be strong enough to carry the extra weight, and this may lead to problems such as bowing (bending) of the bones.

Menstrual problems

Overweight girls tend to enter puberty and begin menstruating earlier than thinner girls. Some complain of more painful menstrual periods. In addition, polycystic ovary syndrome, in which girls may stop menstruating or have irregular periods as well as hirsutism (excess facial or body hair), is associated with being overweight. Other symptoms of this syndrome may include acne, infertility and enlarged ovaries with many small cysts.

Cancer

Studies show that obesity is linked to an increased risk for the development of certain types of cancer, such as stomach and colon cancer, in adults.

Liver problems

Gallbladder disease and liver abnormalities are associated with being overweight. Some people who are overweight develop a chronic condition of the liver with fatty infiltration and inflammation.

Other

Obesity can put one at risk for other medical complications including stroke.

Mortality

Individuals who are obese have an increased risk of death compared with individuals who are of normal weight (Zametkin 2004; National Institute of Diabetes and Kidney Diseases website).

Social and Psychological Problems

Being overweight is not only associated with the medical problems mentioned above. It can affect almost every aspect of a person's life. For some, the effect on their personal and social life is the most devastating of all. Self-esteem suffers. I have had young people tell me that they dreaded going out because people stared at them. Some struggle to find clothes that fit. For a small percentage of overweight people, it feels safer to just stay at home. Some, but by no means all, may develop symptoms of anxiety or depression.

Prejudice

Unfortunately, even though approximately two-thirds of adults are overweight, there is still prejudice against overweight people in the United States. This is especially directed against the most severely obese, and it's hard to believe that the prejudice sometimes even comes from those who are themselves overweight. I recently saw a movie in which the overweight mother of a teenage girl constantly berated her daughter because of her size. She gave her the message that if she would only lose weight, she would be more beautiful and more successful. Luckily in this case, the young girl had a strong sense of self, was able to maintain a good self image, and understood that her worth was not related to how much she weighed. She also saw the irony in the fact that her mother criticized her weight when she herself was overweight. Unfortunately, not everyone is as strong as this young girl was. I have seen teenagers who have felt shamed by their own families, and who have really poor self-esteem.

According to some reports, most overweight young people in our culture suffer from low self-esteem, and many view themselves as less competent socially. Take a moment to think about the television programs you watch and the articles and magazines you read. You have probably seen numerous images of super-muscular men or very thin models, and been inundated with the message that muscular and thin equates with success and beauty. The media have such a powerful influence that it's no wonder if some of you may sometimes feel that you don't measure up. This has got to change. Losing weight should be about becoming healthier and fitter and feeling better, and should not be about changing your appearance to conform to the current popular image.

Teasing and bullying

A study found that overweight teenagers are more likely than those who are not overweight to be involved in bullying. They are more likely to be victims of bullying, but in some cases are the perpetrators. I have had many young people tell me that they are teased or bullied at school. Some fight back, but others just turn away, hoping the bully will go away. Some even switch schools, thinking that their problems will be left behind. Unfortunately, teasing and bullying is still a real problem. If you are being victimized, confide in a parent, teacher or counselor right away. No one should tolerate bullying or teasing. If your friends tease someone else, don't just stand by. Say something! Tell them that this is unacceptable and that you won't be a part of it. This means taking a risk, but you will gain strength and respect in the process. Most people — including your peers — know that bullies are cowards underneath, trying to look strong.

Quality of life

Many young people say that although they are not significantly depressed, being overweight affects their quality of life. They may have more pain, such as lower back or knee pain, which keeps them from participating in physical activities. They may be tired and lack energy to perform tasks at school or work. Some complain of shortness of breath when they take long walks, climb steps or walk uphill. Being severely overweight can even make it difficult to do simple things like putting on socks or tying shoelaces. Teenagers have also told me that they don't enjoy many social activites such as shopping for clothes or swimming because of embarrassment about their size. Altogether, these problems can significantly affect the ability to enjoy life.

Financial Costs

Obesity is very costly, in terms of both illness and money. Direct costs include money spent on diagnosing and treating illnesses related to obesity. Indirect costs are those related to decreased productivity and lost wages of people disabled by obesity or related illness. When direct and indirect costs are combined, obesity and its related disorders cost the United States about $100 billion per year.

In summary, obesity, with its morbidity — medical, psychological and social — and high financial costs, is such an enormous problem that its implications have been compared to that of cigarette smoking. With the decrease in tobacco use in the United States, it appears that the complications of obesity will soon exceed that of smoking.

Benefits of Weight Loss

We have discussed the complications that can arise from being overweight. On the other hand, losing weight can greatly improve your health and well-being:

- You will feel better. If you are overweight, losing even a small amount of weight can make you feel better, give you more energy and boost your confidence.
- You will move better. Losing weight will make it easier to perform day-to-day activities and to be physically active. It's a vicious cycle. The more overweight you are, the more difficult it is to exercise, and this only perpetuates the weight gain. On the other hand, as you lose weight, it becomes easier and more fun to exercise, and this in turn makes it easier to continue to lose weight. Being more active strengthens your heart and your bones, makes you fitter and can even improve your mood.
- You will decrease your risk of developing heart disease, diabetes, high blood pressure and high cholesterol. Exercise can even boost your immune system; people who exercise regularly tend to get fewer illnesses in general.
- You will save money on health care costs. A huge amount of money

is spent on treating obesity and its complications. It is much better to spend the time and money on keeping healthy. "An ounce of prevention is worth a pound of cure!"
• You might even improve your self-esteem by losing weight, becoming healthier and participating in regular physical activity.

The effects of being overweight and sedentary are "bad news" for your physical and emotional health. The good news is that even with small changes, you can greatly improve your health and well-being. You don't need to do everything at once.

6

Body Image
and Self-esteem

Cindy avoided mirrors whenever she could. If she did look in a mirror, she made sure that she saw only her head and shoulders. The last time she saw a reflection of her hips, she hated what she saw. It affected her so much that, after trying on four different outfits to hide her "bottom," she still felt uncomfortable, and decided not to leave the house at all that day. Although Cindy had a healthy body, she saw herself as fat, and began a dangerous cycle of dieting, and later binge eating. Cindy became more and more self-conscious of her body, and isolated from her friends, until she eventually went to her doctor for help.

Body image refers to the way we feel about our bodies and the way we look. Cindy is an example of someone with a negative body image. A negative body image can occur in both males and females. A person who has a negative body image dislikes the way her body looks, and believes that if she only looked better, her entire life would be so much better. Some go even further to believe that the way they look is a reflection of who they are.

As a teenager you are constantly exposed to influences that can have an impact on the way you feel about your body. Magazines portray images of very muscular men and impossibly thin women. Television shows and movies feature leading ladies and leading men who often conform to a certain beauty ideal. Most young people who strive to look like these models and actors are unlikely to achieve their goal, and are more likely to end up frustrated or — even worse — with an eating disorder. We are bombarded with commercials trying to sell diet products, beauty products and exercise equipment. At the same time we are sold the message that we are not good enough as we are. The outcome is that some people may never feel that they measure up, and may feel constant pressure to fit the model. This kind of media exposure and peer pressure can have a powerful effect on your body image.

We all occasionally have negative thoughts about our bodies, but if you believe that your value as a person depends on the way you look, you have a negative body image, and should seek help. Untreated, this could lead to more severe self-esteem issues, unhealthy eating and eating disorders. By learning to respect your body and developing a healthy body image, you will be in a better position to take care of your body, and appreciate all the important qualities you possess as a unique human being.

Do You Have a Negative Body Image?

Answer the following questions.

- Do you worry about what other people think of the way you look?
- Do you feel worse about yourself after seeing photographs of models or watching movies with actors or actresses who conform to a certain beauty ideal?
- Do you believe that if you lose weight all your problems will disappear?
- When you look in the mirror do you usually feel unhappy with what you see?
- Do you often make negative remarks about your body, such as: "I am so fat," or "No one will ever go out with me — I look so bad"?
- Do you feel unworthy as a person because of your weight or the way you look?
- Do you avoid looking in the mirror because of what you see?
- Do you constantly worry about the way you look?

You may have a negative body image if you answered yes to one or two of these questions; you surely do if you answered yes to three or more.

What Influences Your Body Image?

Your body image develops over the years, and can be influenced by a number of things. A few years ago I did a body-image study at a large East Coast university and asked students what factors they believed had played a part in forming their body image. They listed the media, family and friends, teachers and coaches, and old photographs as factors.

Media

One of the strongest influences the students reported was the media. We are exposed to so many cultural messages about appearance — in magazines, on billboards, on television, in movies and in newspapers. When you look at these images of "beautiful" men and women, it is important to remember that they have professionals doing their hair, clothes and make-up, and that their photographs are often airbrushed to look more "perfect." In other words, the images you see are often not realistic at all. Because of the cultural messages they receive, young women tend to equate thinness with beauty, while young men equate being lean and muscular with good looks (but this does vary across cultures). As you become older, you are able to view these messages more critically, but younger people may have more difficulty interpreting their meaning.

If you have low self-esteem in general, you are more likely to have a negative body image, and not have much confidence in either the way you look or in yourself as a person.

Family and friends

Family and friends influence they way we feel about our bodies. You have been influenced by the messages received from your parents and even picked up on messages between your parents. If your father always criticizes your mother for having big thighs, or your mother teases your father about his "fat belly," this may have an effect on the way you see yourself. Friends have a powerful influence too. One woman told me that she will never forget a comment that her friend made to her in her senior year. The exact words were: "I didn't recognize you. Did you gain weight?" Although she was never over-weight, she feels uncomfortable with her body to this day.

Teachers and coaches

Teachers, coaches and trainers can have a strong impact on teenagers in general, and sometimes on the way they feel about themselves and their bodies. I heard of a young girl who loved to dance. She joined a ballet class and was told that she would never become a good dancer unless she became thinner. This was in spite of the fact that she was at a healthy weight. She wanted to excel so badly, that she took the advice and dieted until she reached a dangerously low weight, and could not continue dancing. You've probably heard of boys on the wrestling team having to "make weight" for their category by severely restricting their calories or by "sweating." These are dangerous practices. I'm sure you look up to your teachers and coaches, and it's important that they guide you in a responsible manner. I am happy to say that I have seen most teachers and coaches do a wonderful job.

Pictures

Some students said that looking at old photographs or looking in the mirror affected the way they felt about their bodies. One young girl told me that her first diet was triggered by seeing a photograph of herself at her tenth birthday party.

Puberty

Puberty is a time when young people may be at risk for developing a negative body image. Girls, especially, start developing physical changes that don't correspond to their physical ideal of beauty. They develop more body fat and bigger hips, and those who feel badly about themselves may begin to diet. Girls are not the only ones at risk. Boys are also at risk for developing a negative body image during puberty and adolescence when "fitting in" is so important.

Why Is a Negative Body Image Harmful?

Negative body image and low self-esteem can lead to physical and mental problems, including depression, dangerous dieting behaviors, risk-taking behaviors and eating disorders. Because of this, if you think you may have either of these, it is worth getting help as soon as possible. You can start by contacting your primary-care doctor who will give you a referral if necessary.

Treatment

Treatment for self-esteem issues usually involves some form of counseling, either individually, with your family, or in a group. The therapist will help you explore the causes of the problem, and work on ways in which you can restore your self-esteem and improve your body image. If you are not eating as well as you should, it will be useful also to meet with a dietitian to evaluate your nutrition, and assess any deficiencies.

What Else Can You Do to Prevent a Negative Body Image?

Maintain a healthy lifestyle

Doing some form of regular physical activity is important for your health, can help you feel good about yourself, and can improve your mood. Don't let exercise become an obsession, though; do it in moderation.

Have a good attitude

Instead of having negative thoughts, say or at least think something positive about your body each day. For example, you may say that you are grateful that you have a strong and healthy body, or you may be proud that you can be different instead of fitting a mold.

Don't worry so much about what other people think!

You can't control what they think, and you can't know for sure what they are thinking. On the other hand, you can control what *you* think and what *you* do. Think positive thoughts and you will be happier. By not worrying about what others think of you and the way you look or what you wear, you will be free to concentrate on more important things. Remember that you can never please everybody. The "friend" who said "I didn't recognize you" has a bigger problem than the person she was (thoughtlessly) criticizing.

Do something good for yourself each day

For example, get at least five servings of fruits and vegetables a day, instead of engaging in dangerous behaviors such as very restrictive dieting.

View the media critically

When you watch a movie or television, watch with a critical eye. Ask yourself if the writer or director is trying to "sell" you an idea. Understand that lots of money is put into commercials and ads to sell you on certain ideas or products. Keep away from magazines that promote unhealthy dieting, rapid weight loss, and feature unrealistic images of very thin models.

Keep a journal of your thoughts and feelings

Consider writing down positive thoughts in a journal. Make a note of your accomplishments and the qualities you admire in yourself. This will not make you vain!

Get support

Get support from family and friends, and surround yourself with people you trust and who make you feel good. One of the girls I spoke to said that the way she felt about herself and her body depended upon whom she was with. When she spent time with the girls who berated themselves and were always dieting and fussing about their appearance, she felt negatively about her body, but when she spent time with her good friends, who were more interested in who she was inside, she felt happy about her body and herself.

Don't tolerate teasing or stereotyping on the basis of size and weight

It's demeaning and harmful to your own self-respect as well as to others.

Be thankful for what you have

Eighteen-year-old Jennifer told me the following story:

"Although I didn't complain often, I went through life not really enjoying anything very much. I socialized, but didn't ever feel really comfortable around lots of people. Although I was healthy and not overweight, I was always self-conscious about my body. I thought that my thighs were too big, and that if I were thinner everything would be so much better. So that's how I drifted along, doing what I needed to do, but not putting my heart into anything — and definitely not having fun. Two months ago I had such a scare. My doctor found something wrong on my blood test, and we were afraid that it might be a sign of a serious illness. Further tests had to be done. I had to wait for a whole week until all the test results came back. During that week I was so afraid. I realized how lucky I had been to be healthy up to this point, and to be able to have experienced so many wonderful things. I felt sorry for myself for having to deal with this. I realized that, depending upon those results, everything might change. I started noticing everything around me — the beauty of nature, the ocean, the trees. I wanted to spend more time with the people I loved. How could I ever have worried about whether my thighs were too big? It seemed so trivial now. A week later I was told the good news that I would be okay. I know that experience changed my life. For me it's now about being healthy and strong, not about whether I fit into size four jeans."

The question is sometimes raised about whether girls dress a certain way or feel pressured to look a certain way to impress boys or other girls. Mimi Nichter, an anthropologist who has studied the culture of teenage girls, interviewed them in regard to this subject. They indicated that there was a lot of pressure on girls to look good and to follow certain rules for appropriate dress. Some were afraid that if they didn't follow the "rules" guys would tease them, and some were concerned about being socially rejected by other girls. Think about this for a moment. Do you feel pressured by anyone to look or dress a certain way? Hopefully you will do what feels right and comfortable to you.

7

How Do You Know
If You're Overweight?

Before beginning any treatment plan, you must know whether or not you have a weight problem and determine the extent of the problem. With guidance, you can then plan the program that will suit you best.

Who Can Assess Whether You Are Overweight?

Your primary care doctor

If you or your family are not sure if you have a problem or don't know where to begin, a good place to start is with your pediatrician or family physician. He or she will be able to determine whether your weight is in the normal range, whether you should maintain your weight as you grow in height, or whether you should lose weight. Your doctor can also determine whether there are any associated or underlying problems by doing the following:

- Taking a thorough medical history, including a history of physical activity as well as eating patterns. Your personal history can give clues about any medical problems that may need to be further investigated. Your family history will give information about family members with weight problems, eating disorders or illnesses such as thyroid problems or diabetes.
- Doing a physical examination — sometimes signs of an underlying medical problem can be picked up on examination. For example, if you have thinning hair and a low heart rate and blood pressure, you may have hypothyroidism.

- Measuring your height and weight and evaluating your body mass index, as discussed earlier. Ask your doctor in which percentile your body mass index falls. In children and teenagers, a body mass index at or above the 95th percentile is considered overweight and one between the 85th and 95th percentiles is considered "at risk for becoming overweight."
- Evaluating lab tests to look for causes or complications of obesity, as well as any other medical problems. Lab tests may reveal high blood cholesterol levels, thyroid abnormalities, insulin resistance or diabetes and/or hormone problems, among other things. An electrocardiogram (EKG) and stress test should be done to assess your heart function if you are significantly overweight.
- Evaluating your mental health. A large percentage of young people who are overweight suffer from low self-esteem, and some have depression or anxiety disorders. A significant number have binge-eating disorder, a type of eating disorder.

If treatment is necessary, your doctor can then help with an initial treatment plan or point you in the right direction. Your primary-care physician may feel quite comfortable treating you, perhaps together with a dietitian, or in some cases he or she may refer you to a team more familiar with the treatment of weight problems.

A dietitian

An R.D. (registered dietitian) is an expert on the role of nutrition in health. A registered dietitian has completed at least four years of education in a program approved by the American Dietetic Association. He or she must also complete an internship program and pass an exam to demonstrate knowledge in the field of nutrition. A registered dietitian can evaluate your eating habits, assess any nutritional deficiencies, help you with meal planning, and answer your questions on nutrition. Some people call themselves nutritionists, but they may not necessarily be qualified to give accurate nutrition information. Ask for their credentials.

Who Treats Young People with Weight Problems?

Once they have made the diagnosis, primary-care doctors such as pediatricians or family practitioners often feel comfortable continuing to manage and treat children and teenagers who are overweight. In addition, dietitians can provide consultation and nutritional education. If necessary, therapists can provide individual, family or group therapy to address problems such as binge eating or depression. If a patient suffers from more severe depression or an anxiety disorder, for example, a psychiatrist may sometimes prescribe medication. Young people with weight problems are sometimes referred to a center with a team of healthcare providers, who will address their medical, psychological and nutritional needs.

How Do You Find a Comprehensive Treatment Center?

You can ask for a referral from your primary-care doctor. Your doctor may have a list of resources or should be able to point you in the right direction. You may also receive a referral from the local hospital in your area. Your best bet is to call the teaching hospital nearest you. They may be associated with a treatment center or can give you a referral. A school nurse or counselor may be able to suggest a treatment center, or you may be able to rely on word-of-mouth: it is very reassuring to receive a referral from a satisfied friend. You may find centers listed in the telephone book or on the Internet, and there is also a list of resources at the end of this book.

Is Treatment Covered by Insurance Plans?

The cost of treating obesity is enormous. Unfortunately insurance companies provide very poor coverage for the prevention and treatment of obesity and its related illnesses. I find it ironic that they will often cover the very high costs of obesity surgery, medical complications or hospitalization, and seldom cover the significantly lower costs of early treatment and prevention. I hope that this will change in the near future.

8

Treatment Basics

During adolescence your body is changing rapidly, and to support its growth and development you need adequate calories and essential nutrients. On the other hand, getting too many calories will tip the scale the other way. How do you balance your needs? The number of calories required differs for each person, depending on a number of factors, such as age, sex, growth, and metabolic rate. It will also vary depending on how active you are. Check with your doctor or a dietitian to get an idea of what you need. If you are tempted to go on a very-low-calorie diet, don't! Drastically cutting down on calories to lose weight can lead to serious health problems, including thinning of your bones, heart problems and eating disorders. Your body may slow its metabolic rate in response to greatly reduced intake, making further weight loss progressively more difficult. Making gradual healthy changes can result in a lifetime of healthier nutrition, a healthy weight and a healthy body.

As you develop your plan, remember that overweight is a health concern, not a cosmetic one. In other words, the primary reason for losing weight if you are overweight should be to improve your health and prevent complications associated with obesity, not to change your appearance. Of course there are many other benefits that come from losing weight, such as increased energy, better self-esteem, and improvement in quality of life. If you concentrate on striving toward healthier eating and some form of regular physical activity, the rest will follow.

The key to permanent weight loss is to find a long-term safe plan that you can follow always. The reason that few people are able to maintain their weight loss is that they diet and lose weight, and then return to their old habits, only to regain the weight they lost or more.

Avoid restrictive diets. Instead eat balanced meals and snacks, and remain physically active, to become strong and fit. Think in terms of lifelong changes that you can live with, rather than in terms of a short-term quick fix.

We know that making changes in lifestyle behaviors and long-term habits isn't easy, but because of the serious problems that can result from being overweight, it is definitely worth the effort. Unfortunately, until recently, doctors and other healthcare providers were reluctant to address the problem of overweight and obesity. Some were uncomfortable talking about such a sensitive issue. Many had too little time or they were pessimistic about the outcome of treatment. I have heard some doctors say they were afraid that treatment of obesity would lead to eating disorders. In spite of these concerns, however, it is clear that we have to do something about this growing problem.

What Do You Do First?

Once you know you need to lose weight, you need to form a plan of action.

- First make a commitment to becoming healthier and fitter. When you are sufficiently motivated to make a change, it will happen.
- Before beginning a serious weight-loss or exercise program, discuss this with your doctor.
- Work together with your doctor or a registered dietitian to set realistic goals for yourself. Write them down. If you envision your goals, you are more likely to reach them. Aim to reach a healthy weight by making small changes—one at a time. Gradually begin to eat more nutritiously and slowly start increasing your physical activity. Weight-loss goals will differ from person to person, and will depend on whether you are still growing in height. A reasonable initial goal might be to lose between one and four pounds a month. It's usually not a good idea for young people to lose weight

much faster than this. Setting both short-term and long-term goals will help to keep you more motivated. For example, set a goal to take a twenty-minute walk at least three days a week. Reward yourself if you achieve the goal, and then set your next goal. Don't be too hard on yourself if you don't always reach your goals. Try a little harder the next time, or re-evaluate your goals to see whether they are realistic.

- If you live at home, involve your family to the extent that you are able and feel comfortable. It's much easier if the whole family commits to a healthier lifestyle.
- Don't expect a quick fix. It's not the best way to do this! It is far better to take small steps and make lasting changes, rather than lose weight rapidly only to regain it soon after.

Do you know that even if you are severely overweight, even a small amount of weight loss (5 percent or 10 percent of your body weight) can improve your health significantly?

What Motivates You?

You hold the power to change. No one can force you to live a healthy lifestyle. However, if you make up your mind that you want to make a change, you can do it. You'll have a much easier time if you're motivated — in other words, if you're really driven by a strong desire to change, for whatever reason. Take some time to think of what motivates you, because not everyone has the same motivation, even when it comes to weight loss and fitness. Could it be:

Your health

You may want to lose weight to become healthier, or to prevent disease. There has certainly been so much written about the complications of being overweight, with the increased risk for problems such as high cholesterol, high blood pressure, and diabetes. You may even have someone in your family with one of these illnesses, and therefore be more concerned. One of the teenage boys I interviewed was entirely motivated by health reasons. His uncle had high cholesterol and had developed heart disease. He learned that his uncle's health problems would have been prevented by a healthier lifestyle.

Fitness/sports

Your motivation may be wanting to become fitter to be able to participate in a particular sport, for example to make the track team, or the basketball team, or to improve your athletic ability in general. A thirteen-year-old girl told me that she began eating more healthily and working out regularly in order to become a better soccer player.

Appearance

You may want to lose weight to change your appearance. Teenagers have told me that they felt that people treated them differently because they were overweight, and others told me that it was extremely difficult to find nice clothes that fit. Some girls avoid going to the mall with their friends because they are embarrassed to try on clothes. Maybe you're motivated to lose weight because you feel that you'll be more accepted by your friends. If this is your only motivation, I ask you to think about weight loss in a different way. Sure, your appearance will change, and you may find it easier to buy clothes, but weight loss should never be all about appearance. It's really about a healthier life.

For someone else

Quite often, when I ask a young girl or boy why they came to my office, they tell me that one of their parents "made them come in for treatment." They tell me that they are doing this just for their parents, and that they don't themselves have any interest in changing.

To feel better

There are so many benefits to losing weight and becoming fitter, besides the obvious health benefits. Overweight people who lose weight have more energy, move better, and just feel better overall. You may be fed up with having no energy, finding it difficult to move around quickly and dealing with aching feet and aching joints. You may be motivated by wanting a better quality of life. After losing even a small amount of weight, you will probably feel better, and this may motivate you to continue your healthier lifestyle.

A friend's success

One teenage boy told me that he was motivated by his best friend who had lost a lot of weight, and was now feeling so much better physically and mentally. He believed that if his friend could succeed, so could he.

The challenge

Some people enjoy challenging themselves. They see it as a challenge to be able to achieve weight loss and fitness. They set goals for themselves and are motivated by proving to themselves that they can reach their goals. What better challenge can there be than challenging yourself to become healthier?

You may have other reasons for wanting to lose weight. It's up to you to figure out what motivates you. I'll tell you that if you're doing it for yourself, rather than only to please someone else, it's much more powerful.

What Is Standing in Your Way?

Let's say you've decided that you need to lose weight, and you've worked out what motivates you. Yet it's still hard to take the next step — to actually do anything about it. Why? There are many possible things that can stand in the way of reaching your goals. Figure out what's been stopping you, and you're more likely to be successful. Below are some problems that can stand between you and a healthy, fit lifestyle.

No time

Often I hear from teenagers that they don't have time to eat healthily and exercise. Believe me, I know how busy your life is. I understand that you have to get up early in the morning, and rush to be on time for school. After school, you have homework and perhaps after-school activities. You've also got to fit in some social life, and you probably have chores to do around the house. This book is for you. It requires making gradual, simple changes that can fit into almost any schedule. It takes only a small amount of planning, and as your new way of life becomes habit, it gets easier and easier.

Wrong information

There is a lot of conflicting information out there. It's sometimes difficult to know what to do to be healthy. First you read that you should go on a low-fat diet, then you hear that "carbs" are bad for you. Then you worry about trans-fats. On top of this, there are so many books trying to sell the latest fad diet. Not having the right information can stand in the way of a healthy lifestyle.

Illness

Illnesses such as depression, or binge-eating disorder (a type of eating disorder) can make it more difficult for you to lose weight on your own. It's important that you seek professional help.

Fear of change

Some people are truly afraid of changing, afraid even of losing weight. They may be afraid of the unknown if they've always been overweight, or they may hold on to their extra weight as a form of "protection," a way of distancing themselves from other people. One young man told me that even though he was unhappy with his weight, it was easier to keep doing what he had always done, than to face change.

Sabotage

You may be doing everything you know how to do to become healthier, but there may be someone undermining your efforts. Perhaps you have a neighbor who constantly brings you tempting cakes, or you may have a friend who feels threatened by your weight-loss attempts and urges you to eat more. Some people eat because they don't want to hurt others' feelings.

Lack of resources and support

Maybe you don't have access to resources such as a gym. Perhaps you live in a neighborhood without parks or sidewalks and find it difficult or unsafe to take walks in your area. You may also not have the support you would like, from family and friends. On the other hand, family members may want to be supportive, but may not know how. They may even be struggling with their own weight and health issues.

All of these obstacles can be overcome, and I will cover these circumstances throughout the book. Knowing what's standing in your way of achieving better health, can be the first step to overcoming it.

What Does Treatment Involve?

If you go to a healthcare provider or a center dealing with weight issues, your treatment will probably involve some combination of the following:

- Working together with your healthcare provider to find ways to improve your nutrition and increase your physical activity.
- Teaching you how to modify your behaviors to help develop life-long healthier habits and life skills. You will learn how to set goals and monitor yourself, and how to replace unhealthy behaviors with healthier ones.
- Treating any existing medical problems.
- Psychotherapy. Not everyone who needs to lose weight needs therapy, but in certain situations it can be very helpful. Therapy can improve self-esteem, relationships, and help with binge eating. Therapists can also deal with problems such as depression or anxiety. Therapy may be individual, family or group.
- Treating associated psychiatric problems with medication if necessary.
- Medications. Sometimes drugs are used (in addition to lifestyle

changes) to treat obesity. However, results have not been very encouraging, and medications have side-effects and can be expensive. Medication such as metformin may be used in the case of insulin resistance or diabetes. Also, there are other medications that, although they have not been formally approved to treat obesity, have been used for people with binge eating. Most of the time, though, medication is not needed when treating someone who is overweight.
• Surgery for obesity is rarely an option in children and teenagers, and is outside the scope of this book.

Most young people will do well simply by improving their nutrition and increasing their physical activity. These are the keys to becoming healthier and fitter.

9

Healthy Nutrition: The First Step in Change

When you take in more energy (calories) than you use up, you gain weight. To lose weight, you need to burn off more calories (energy) than you eat. That sounds simple, doesn't it? But in practice, as you probably know, it's not that simple. For some people, counting calories can be boring and time-consuming, and for others it may become an obsession. Also, people vary greatly in their nutritional needs, so one "diet" does not fit all. Last but not least, people eat for many reasons other than hunger, so addressing only their calorie needs will not be enough: emotional needs also play a role.

Decreasing caloric intake and increasing physical activity are the basic and essential elements of successful weight loss, so we will discuss how you achieve this without having to obsess about how many calories you eat each day.

To lose weight safely you need to decrease the total number of calories you take in each day, while maintaining a balanced diet. A good, balanced eating plan is very important if you want to become healthier and lose weight permanently. Although physical activity is an essential part of a healthy lifestyle, if you want to lose a significant amount of weight, you will also have to modify your eating habits. The good news is that in order to be successful, you don't have to go hungry and you never have to feel deprived: see the section "Look at what you can eat!" Even if you do need to lose a large amount of weight, losing it in a slow and steady manner is still safest. Your weight loss is more likely to be permanent if it's gradual.

Nutrition Basics

It's worth having some understanding of food labels. Food labels can be useful to compare brands of products, or to make you aware of which foods are higher in fat, or to give you an idea of fiber content, for example. They should be only a guide, though. Many pre-packaged foods will now contain detailed nutritional information. Even some restaurants are now making the nutritional content of their menu items available. A quick look at calories, fat and carbohydrate content, as well as grams of fiber, will tell you much of what you need to know. The ingredient list tells you what's in the food, and lists ingredients in descending order. If sugar is at the top of the list, it is not a food that should be eaten frequently. You must remember, however, that the nutritional information given is that contained in one serving size, and serving sizes are often smaller than many people imagine. A soda may contain 90 calories per serving, but if the bottle contains two servings, you will be drinking 180 calories if you finish the soda. Be aware that some packages of snack foods may contain several servings, so if you plan on eating only one serving, think hard whether you really want to buy the whole bag. Once you get an idea of the nutritional content of the foods you frequently eat, you will know which foods are healthier for you, and you will be more aware of appropriate portions. Soon you'll find that you won't need to spend as much time reading food labels.

Calories

Losing weight comes down to how many calories you take in, and how many calories you burn off. A question I often get asked is: "How many calories do I need each day?" Your energy (calorie) needs vary depending on your metabolism, your age and sex, and how active you are, among other factors. It would be neither fair nor accurate to give you an exact number. Your doctor or a dietitian can help you determine your specific calorie needs.

To illustrate a point, however, let's say you want to lose a pound of weight in a week. Because a pound is equivalent to 3,500 calories, you have to take in 500 fewer calories a day, burn off 500 more calories a day, or combine these two approaches, in order to lose that pound. The easiest would be to combine the two: for example, take in 200 fewer calories a day, and burn off 300 more a day. By decreasing the amount you eat a little, and by increasing your physical activity, it will be easier to achieve your goal.

I mentioned this to give you some idea of what it takes to lose weight. I don't recommend that you count calories on a daily basis. As I indicated before, it's not practical, it can lead to obsessiveness, and some even say it takes the fun out of eating. (Eating is something that should be enjoyed!) Instead, if you eat balanced meals with plenty of nutritious foods, get enough fiber in your diet, and do regular physical activity, you will find that you don't have to count calories.

In this book you will learn ways of eating that will naturally promote a lower intake of calories. For example, we know that filling up on healthy, low-calorie foods will leave less room for high-calorie, high-fat foods. So, starting a meal with a green salad, fresh fruit or a bowl of broth-based or vegetable soup will fill you so that you will probably eat fewer calories during your meal. It is rare for anyone to become fat on fruits and vegetables, so feel free to eat plenty of them! Eat slowly: hunger decreases only when nutrients are absorbed. It takes at least 20 minutes for the food you have eaten to "register" with your brain.

You will also learn ways to increase your physical activity. If you are not very active, adding even half an hour of physical activity on a few days a week will burn off hundreds of extra calories. As long as you don't compensate by eating more, you'll soon see and feel the positive results.

Portions

Remember the saying: "Too much of a good thing..."? If you eat too much of even a good food, you will probably gain weight. Apart from being more inactive, another reason Americans are gaining weight is that they are eating larger portion sizes. To give you an idea: The United States Department of Agriculture (USDA) standard serving size for meat is 3 oz. and some restaurants offer servings of anywhere from 7 oz. to over 30 oz.! When I moved to the United States in 1983, I was shocked by the size of restaurant hamburgers and sandwiches here. Fast-food restaurants offer larger sizes of sodas, burgers and fries, and we have become quite accustomed to these bigger sizes.

If you eat fast foods it's important that you have some idea of their nutritional value. Let me give you an idea of the calorie and fat content of some of the popular fast foods. See how the smaller-sized version compares to the larger size. A McDonald's hamburger provides 280 calories and 10 grams of fat. Compare this to a Double Quarter Pounder with cheese that has 770 calories and 47 grams of fat. A small order of French fries has 230 calories and 11 grams of fat, while a Super Size serving has 610 calories and 29 grams of fat (almost three times the amount). Because we have become so accustomed to large portion sizes, we are starting to serve these larger sizes at home too.

When people are offered larger portions, they tend to eat more. When we open a large bag of chips, or buy a larger carton of movie popcorn, we will probably eat more than we would out of a small bag. When offered a large plate of food, the tendency is to eat more than one would off a small plate of food. Also, although a plate of meat or fish with a salad and vegetables is a healthy meal, some people forget that having a second serving of even a healthy food doubles the calories and may provide more than is really needed for a meal.

Eat slowly, and then decide (no sooner than 15 or 20 minutes after starting the meal) whether you really need that second serving. If you still are hungry, go for it. Play a friendly trick on your eyes and your stomach by using a smaller plate when helping yourself to food. Also, buy snacks in small single-serving packages. That way you will be less tempted to eat more than you really want to eat. A simple rule of thumb for a balanced dinner is as follows: imagine your plate divided into four quarters. Fill one quarter with a protein, such as fish, chicken or meat. Fill the second quarter with a starch such as brown rice or potato (preferably sweet potato). Fill the last two quarters with two or more vegetables such as broccoli, beans, carrots or squash. Feel free to have a green salad with a low-fat dressing or a fruit and/or a serving of low-fat yogurt on the side. Remember to drink plenty of water.

In summary then, by choosing smaller portions, avoiding second servings, and buying snacks in single-serving sizes, you will automatically cut down on your calories without having to count them.

WHAT IS A SERVING SIZE?

The following are examples of single serving sizes:

- 3 ounces of meat (the size of a deck of cards)
- 1 medium-sized fruit such as a banana or an apple
- a quarter-cup of dried fruit
- a half-cup of vegetables
- a half-cup of cooked pasta
- 1 slice of bread
- 1 cup of milk or yogurt (choose low-fat or fat-free milk if possible)
- a half-cup of frozen yogurt or ice cream
- 2 tablespoons of peanut butter

Dietary fats

Believe it or not, although fats did get a bad name in the past, they make up an important part of a healthy diet. They have many necessary functions, including helping in the production of hormones in the body and helping with the transport of fat-soluble vitamins— A, D, E and K. Of course you don't want to overdo it, as they contain more calories per gram (9 per gram) than do proteins and carbohydrates, and so you can more easily gain weight when you eat too much fat. You may also gain more weight from eating fat because fat does not seem to be as filling or satisfy hunger as well as proteins and carbohydrates do, and so the tendency is to eat more.

Some people argue that Americans have gained weight despite lowering the percentage of fat in their diets during the "low-fat" craze. Although this may be true, it's misleading. What probably happened was the following: although the fat percentage in the American diet did go down after 1970, for many their total calories increased as did their actual fat intake.

About 30 percent of your total calories should come from fats. Fats such as mono- and poly-unsaturated fats are healthier than saturated fats. Saturated fats can raise your blood cholesterol and should be limited to 10 percent of your daily calories. Although the percentage of fat in a food may appear to be low, the total number of fat grams and total calorie content many still be significant, so read the label. For example, whole milk has 3.5 percent fat but 8 grams of fat and 150 calories in one cup. In comparison, reduced-fat milk (2 percent fat) has 5 grams of fat and about 120 calories, and a cup of skim milk has 0 grams of fat and 90 calories. Trans fats or trans fatty acids can be found naturally or are created by adding hydrogen to unsaturated fats to make food last longer. These hydrogenated oils can increase one's risk for heart disease. It's therefore best to reduce your intake of trans fats in processed foods. The above is only a guide. A dietitian can easily assess what you eat and give you an idea of whether the amount of fat you take in is reasonable. Below are a few examples of foods containing the different types of fats:

- Saturated fats—Butter, cheese, coconut or coconut oil, palm oil, vegetable shortening, and the skin on poultry.
- Mono-unsaturated fats—cashew nuts, peanuts, olives, olive oil.
- Poly-unsaturated fats—almonds, fish, safflower oil, soybean oil.
- Trans fats—found in many fast foods, chips, cookies, pastries and some margarines.

You can decrease your intake of fat by choosing lower-fat alternatives. Compare the following salad dressings for example: a serving of creamy caesar dressing can provide up to 190 calories and 18 grams of fat. A lower-fat alternative is a low-fat balsamic vinaigrette which has 40 calories and only 3 grams of fat per serving. You can also cut your fat intake by grilling, baking or broiling, instead of frying, and by choosing lean meats and removing the skin from chicken before cooking.

So, you shouldn't eliminate fats, because some fat is necessary in your diet, but it's best to favor foods containing unsaturated fats rather than saturated fats.

Cholesterol

There are two main types of cholesterol in the blood-stream. Low-density lipoprotein (LDL), also known as "bad" cholesterol, deposits fat and cholesterol (plaques) on the walls of arteries, narrowing them and restricting blood flow. On the other hand, high-density lipoprotein (HDL), or "good" cholesterol, removes fat and cholesterol from artery walls and may prevent heart disease. Most of the cholesterol in your blood is made by your liver and the rest comes from the food you eat. Cholesterol occurs in foods such as meats, eggs, milk and other dairy products.

Carbohydrates

Carbohydrates are an essential part of a healthy nutrition plan. They make up 50–60 percent of the calories in the average American diet, and provide our primary source of energy. Diets that call for eliminating carbohydrates make no sense. Your body converts carbohydrates into glucose, which is converted into energy. The main carbohydrates are sugars and starches. Sugar is found naturally in some foods such as fruits (fructose) and milk (lactose), and is added to other foods and drinks such as candy, pastries, processed foods and soft drinks, to make them taste sweet. Complex carbohydrates or starches are made up of sugars linked together. They include foods such as grains, peas, beans and potatoes. Starches need more time to digest, and make one feel full longer.

Even though carbohydrates contain fewer calories than does an equivalent amount of fat, 4 versus 9 calories for every gram, "fat-free" does not mean calorie-free. "No-calorie" diet sodas, for example, use artificial sweeteners instead of sugar. Many fat-free foods are loaded with sugars to make them taste better. They may have just as many calories as the fat-free version, and may sometimes have more. Reduced-fat peanut butter has the same calorie load as the regular variety. When you read food labels, be aware that sugars may be hidden in the ingredients under a different name, such as corn syrup, high-fructose corn syrup, maltose or dextrose, for example.

You don't need to avoid carbohydrates, but favor complex carbohydrates, and limit your intake of refined carbohydrates such as white rice, white bread and other white-flour products. Instead choose whole-grain cereals, whole-wheat breads and whole-wheat-flour products.

Protein

Protein — 4 calories per gram — helps with the growth and repair of cells in the body, and can be used as a source of energy when carbohydrates and fat are insufficient. Although it's important to get adequate amounts of protein during adolescence, it is rare for teenagers in the United States to become deficient in protein. Protein can be derived from numerous sources, such as meat, fish, soybeans, milk products, eggs, or dried beans and peas.

Alcohol

Alcohol, which is not an essential nutrient, falls into a separate category from proteins, carbohydrates or fats. It is processed by the liver and stored as fat. Alcohol provides more calories per gram than either carbohydrates or protein (7 versus 4). Drinking alcohol (beer or wine) can also stimulate appetite. So, not only is alcohol intake illegal for teenagers, it can also contribute to excessive weight gain.

Fiber (roughage)

Fiber, made up of components of plant materials, provides bulk in food and helps you feel fuller even with fewer calories. It provides almost no calories because it is mostly not digested. People tend to lose more weight when, in addition to choosing low-fat foods, they add more fiber to their diets. Fiber is found in fruits and vegetables, whole grains, beans and peas. Fresh fruits and vegetables are an excellent choice, but frozen fruits and vegetables and dried fruits are good alternatives. There are two types of fiber. Insoluble fiber, also known as "roughage," allows food to travel through the intestines more quickly. It does not dissolve in water. Examples of insoluble fiber include whole grains and vegetables. Soluble fiber dissolves in water and has been shown to slow down digestion, and to decrease serum cholesterol. Soluble fiber is found in beans, fruits and oat products. Studies show that populations that have a higher intake of fiber and complex carbohydrates tend to be less overweight.

Let's now review how many calories each of the following nutrients provides for every gram:

- Fat — 9 calories
- Carbohydrate — 4 calories
- Protein — 4 calories
- Alcohol — 7 calories

The Food Pyramid

The United States Department of Agriculture has developed a "food pyramid" that serves as a guide to the kinds and quantities of foods you should eat on a daily basis. It can help you make sure you get the balance of nutrients that you need. The pyramid is divided into various food groups and lists the number of servings recommended for each group.

Vitamin and Mineral Supplements

It is probably not necessary to take a daily vitamin or mineral supplement if you're healthy and eat a balanced diet. You may need supplements if you are a vegetarian, are on a very restrictive diet, have an eating disorder or chronic illness, or don't eat dairy products.

Vitamins

Although you need a variety of vitamins for normal growth and development, the foods you eat will usually provide you with these. Under certain circumstances, such as those listed above, you may be prescribed vitamin supplements.

Minerals

A balanced diet is important to ensure that you get an adequate amount of minerals, including calcium, iron and zinc.

Many teenagers don't get the recommended amount of calcium, about 1,200 to 1,500 milligrams per day. Today teenagers are drinking more soft drinks and juices and less calcium-rich milk. Calcium is necessary for normal bone development. If you don't get enough calcium in your diet, you are at risk for developing osteoporosis ("thinning of the bones"). Taking in too much phosphorus by drinking too many carbonated sodas may play a role in increasing your risk further. Besides protecting against osteoporosis, recent studies also suggest that calcium in low-fat or non-fat dairy products may even help you lose weight. Be sure that you get the calcium you need by taking in adequate amounts of low-fat milk or other dairy products, dark-green leafy vegetables, or canned salmon or sardines (with bones). If you don't think you are getting enough calcium in your diet, ask your doctor whether you need a calcium supplement.

Iron deficiency is the most common nutritional deficiency in the United States. Make sure that you are getting enough iron in your diet. Girls can become iron-deficient from loss of iron through menstruation. Teenage boys are at risk near their peak growth period when their iron stores may not meet their growth demands. You can get iron from red meats and green vegetables, but also from other foods such as iron-fortified cereals and dried fruits.

Zinc is a mineral that is important for normal growth and development and healthy skin. You may not be getting enough zinc in your diet if you are vegetarian, so check with your doctor or with a dietitian to see whether you need any supplementation.

Liquids

Water

Make sure you stay hydrated by drinking plenty of plain water every day, especially on hot days or days when you are more physically active. Students often don't get enough to drink during the school day, or they may drink sodas, juices, coffee or tea instead of mostly water. Water provides fluid without unnecessary sugar, carbonation or caffeine. If you are allowed, carry a plastic bottle of water in your backpack as a reminder to drink more water. Drink water *before* you become very thirsty.

Caffeine

Americans consume a lot of caffeine. You'll find a coffee shop almost everywhere you look. Caffeine, which is found in coffee, tea, sodas, chocolate and some medications, is a mild stimulant that can be habit-forming. People often use caffeine because it makes them feel more alert temporarily. However, too much caffeine can lead to problems including restlessness, jitteriness and withdrawal headaches. Instead of using caffeine to stay awake, it's best to eat balanced meals, do regular physical activity and get enough sleep.

Vegetarian or Vegan Diets

A vegetarian is someone who eats mostly fruits, vegetables, grains, nuts and seeds, and may or may not eat dairy products and eggs. Vegans avoid all meat products, eggs and dairy products. Vegetarian and vegan diets provide lots of healthy foods, but may be lacking in iron and other nutrients. If you are a vegetarian or a vegan, check with your doctor or a dietitian to see whether you need a supplement.

Avoid Extremes

Forget the "crash diet" mentality. How many times have you said to yourself: "I'll start my diet next month" or "I'll eat this one last donut, then on Monday, I will start my diet." That's asking for failure. And have you ever told yourself you would never eat sweets or chocolate again, and after a few days of managing to stay away from them, given in to your craving and splurged on all the candy you could get your hands on? Diets are unpleasant and frustrating. They don't work, and they can be dangerous. But you may say: "I know someone who lost a lot of weight on a low-carb diet," or "My friend lost weight on a diet that excluded almost all fats." Sure, you will lose weight on any diet that drastically restricts calories, but this weight loss is usually short-lived — and you will often have to pay a high price for it.

Why is dieting a problem?

If you forbid yourself to eat certain foods you like, you will probably develop cravings for that food, and run the risk of giving in to those cravings and bingeing on the forbidden food. If you restrict your calorie intake too severely, you will have less energy and poor concentration. You may also develop obsessive thinking about food. Diets that are too restrictive can lead to medical problems including muscle weakness, dizziness and fainting, heart problems, osteoporosis, menstrual problems and eating disorders. Extreme dieting can also lead to symptoms of depression and anxiety.

Fad diets

Fad diets are "popular" diets that recommend unusual eating patterns, which are often unbalanced, have no scientific basis, and may be harmful. Children and teenagers may be at greater risk for developing problems from going on such diets. Fad diets do sell books, but they are unlikely to make you healthier or thinner in the long run.

Beware of diets such as the following:

- All-you-can-eat diets.
- Diets that allow very limited foods only, e.g. a grapefruit diet, a cabbage soup diet.
- Diets that recommend only certain combinations of foods.
- Diets that promise very rapid weight loss.
- Crash diets.
- Diets requiring certain supplements, especially when you need to buy them from the person recommending the diet (check with your doctor first).
- Diets that eliminate fruits and vegetables.

- Any short-term "diet" such as a seven-day diet or a one-month diet, that implies that you will come off it at some time. Healthy eating should last a lifetime.
- Diets that require skipping meals.
- Diets that completely eliminate whole food groups. There was a time when very-low-fat diets were popular, and then the craze became "low-carb." Neither extreme is healthy. One needs a balance of all nutrients—proteins, carbohydrates and fats.

Can you believe that Americans spend more than $40 billion a year on dieting and diet-related products? Statistics from the National Eating Disorders Association show this to be true.

Look at What You Can Eat on a Healthy Plan!

When you eat healthily, you don't have to feel deprived. Stop thinking about all the foods you won't be able to eat. Instead, think of all the delicious foods you can eat. Also there's no need to ban any food forever. An occasional sweet treat is fine. Why don't you look forward to a lifetime of eating more healthily rather than eating "perfectly"? You will discover all the wonderful foods and flavors that are not only good for you but also taste good. A healthy nutrition plan includes lots of fruits and vegetables, such as berries, mangoes, oranges, apples, bananas, carrots, beans, peas and salads. It includes chicken, lean meats and fish, as well as vegetarian dishes with tofu, lentils and seeds in salads, chili and stews. You can have whole-grain bread, brown rice and even whole-wheat pasta, and choose from a variety of high-fiber cereals and oats. You will be able to eat low-fat dairy products such as yogurts, milk and cheeses. There will be many choices for healthy snacks, for example low-fat popcorn, dried fruits, frozen yogurts, nuts and raisins. Go for a wide variety of foods, and experiment with new foods so that you will not become bored. You won't be missing much with so many great-tasting options available.

The following are some examples of higher-calorie foods with lower-calorie alternatives. Learn how to make good choices.

- Choose a half-cup of nonfat frozen yogurt that contains about 110 to 140 calories over a half-cup of Ben & Jerry's chocolate chip cookie dough ice cream which contains 300 calories.
- If you want a sandwich, choose turkey (average 30 calories per ounce) over salami (average 80 calories per ounce)
- Choose pretzels (100 calories per ounce) rather than potato chips (150 calories per ounce)
- If you have a craving for something sweet, consider a frozen fruit bar instead of candy, and if you want a salty snack, choose air-popped or low-fat popcorn rather than buttered popcorn.
- Make oven-baked fries instead of traditional French fries. You can do this by putting strips of potato into the oven with some seasoning and a small amount of olive oil.
- Consider a pita with hummus, four whole-wheat crackers with cheese or peanut butter, or a handful of almonds as an afternoon snack. Although nuts and cheese do provide fat (with more calories per gram than protein or carbs) eating these in moderation can help reduce hunger.
- Be creative by adding berries or bananas to cereals and yogurt or enjoying your fruit in a fruit smoothie. Make your own trail mix with raisins, almonds and high-fiber cereal.

Although there are so many more high-fat, sugary snacks available today, we also have more healthy options available to us.

Metabolism

You may blame your metabolism if you can't lose weight easily, but chances are that you have a normal metabolism. "Basal metabolism" or "basal metabolic rate" is the rate at which your body uses up energy to maintain only its basic life processes. This does not take into account how active you are. If you are struggling to lose weight, speak to your doctor about having your basal metabolism checked by a procedure known as "indirect calorimetry." This is done by assessing your resting metabolic rate and determining how many calories you need each day just to perform basic functions such as breathing. Once your activity level is taken into account, healthcare providers can calculate how many calories you need every day either to maintain weight or to lose weight. Of course, if you find out that your resting metabolic rate is normal, you will no longer be able to blame your weight on your metabolism! By the way, even if you do have a normal metabolism, you can speed it up by exercising. Apart from all the other benefits of exercising, it will become easier to lose weight.

"Nutrition in a Nutshell"

What to do

Discuss your nutrition and calorie needs with your doctor or dietitian and set goals for yourself. Remember that if you want to lose a pound a week, you will have to decrease your daily calories by 500, increase your physical activity, or — better still — do a combination of both. You don't have to count every calorie you eat. Instead it's enough to have an approximate idea of how many calories you need.

Eat breakfast every day. If you are not doing so, I think that this is one of the most important changes you can make.

Be aware of portions and serving sizes, and learn how to interpret food labels so that you can make healthier choices.

Modify your behaviors. For example, plan your meals and snacks in advance, if you won't be eating at home. Then, before you reach for a snack, decide whether you are really hungry, or whether you are eating because you are bored, stressed, sad or lonely. If you are unsure, do something else for five minutes, and then if you still want that snack, have it. When you eat meals, eat slowly. You will enjoy your food more, and it takes time to register that you are full. Also, start some of your meals with a low-calorie salad or soup, so that you will be less likely to overeat during the rest of your meal. You can make your environment more health-friendly by limiting temptations. Instead of keeping cookies on the kitchen counter, leave baskets of your favorite fruits.

Limit your intake of fats to approximately 30 percent of your total daily calories and your saturated fat to approximately 10 percent of your daily calories. A dietitian can help you with this.

Choose complex carbohydrates such as brown rice and whole-grain products instead of refined carbohydrates such as white rice and white-flour products.

Make sure that you get enough fiber in your diet. Eating whole grains and at least five servings of fruits and vegetables a day will help you do so. Have plenty of fresh fruits and vegetables around all the time.

Make sure that you get enough calcium in your diet. You can get calcium from low-fat milk, cheese or yogurt. Calcium is essential for strong bones and appears to play a role in weight control.

Drink plenty of water. It is far better for you than drinks containing caffeine or sugar.

Be creative. Healthy foods should still taste good. Experiment with flavors and spices. If your parents do the cooking, ask them to do so. Offer to help sometimes.

Work with your doctor or a dietitian to make healthy nutritional changes—only one or two at a time.

What Not to Do

Don't skip meals. Instead, eat at regular times to avoid becoming so hungry that you develop cravings or begin binge eating. You are more likely to make healthy choices if you are not too hungry.

Keep away from fad diets and very restrictive diets. There are so many of them, in part because they don't work in the long run. They are also usually not safe. Although you may lose weight on a very restrictive diet, it will be difficult to maintain your weight loss, and you may begin to obsess about the foods you have eliminated. I have seen many patients come into my office after having been on fad diets or crash diets, only to regain the weight they lost and more.

Don't give up if your progress is slow at first. It takes time to develop new habits. Unfortunately, some people resort to harmful measures such as smoking or taking pills to try to control their weight. These can have serious consequences. Don't take any weight-loss pills or supplements without the recommendation of your physician, as some of these supplements, such as those containing ephedra, may be harmful to you.

Jim's Story

Jim, a twenty-one-year-old who used to smoke a pack of cigarettes a day, has now quit and says he feels so much better. At first he began to smoke because his friends smoked. He then had the idea that if he smoked more he would eat less and might lose weight. "Soon I realized that this was counterproductive to my weight loss plans," Jim told me. "To maintain a healthy weight and stay fit, I knew I had to be physically active. I couldn't participate in sports while I was smoking regularly. I felt lethargic and out of breath often, and even used to cough up phlegm sometimes. I was also less motivated to get up and do anything physical. Smoking was my crutch." I asked Jim what made him quit smoking. " My girlfriend made me quit. She didn't like what it was doing to my health. She also didn't like the way my clothes smelled. It was very difficult but I'm glad I was able to stop. I am stronger and fitter now. I also have less chance of getting lung cancer."

Learn More

You can learn some basic facts about nutrition in books or by consulting with a registered dietitian. Despite apparent confusion in the literature, a registered dietitian can provide guidance on optimal nutrition, and will help you make sense of it all. A dietitian will be able to create a meal plan for you that balances proteins, carbohydrates and fat, and still allows you to lose weight.

10

Physical Activity: The Second Step

Physical activity is a critical part of a weight-loss program. Regular physical activity plays an important role in your general health and conditioning and can help you keep your weight down. When a large group of people who had successfully kept their weight off for years were interviewed, it was found that the one thing they had in common was regular exercise.

Exercise strengthens your bones and your muscles including your heart muscle, improves your circulation, increases flexibility, helps prevent disease by boosting your immune system, and can help you live longer. It gives you energy, increases self-esteem, can help you concentrate and can improve your mood. It has even been shown to improve academic performance! Exercise also boosts your metabolism, and this in turn helps you lose weight. Weight-bearing exercise can help prevent osteoporosis. How many medications do you know that can provide all this? There aren't any! Begin with a small amount of physical activity, and gradually increase the time and intensity when you are ready. I'm sure you'll feel the benefits.

The new guidelines for physical activity include about sixty minutes per day on most days for healthy individuals. I know this may sound overwhelming to some of you. Don't let this put you off exercising. Remember that if you have not been doing much activity, any increase will be beneficial. I don't recommend that anyone start out with sixty minutes a day. Start with a few minutes of light activity, and gradually increase time and intensity as you are able. Don't do more than you are ready to do. It's not worth risking an injury, which could prevent you from exercising for a long time. If you are a beginner, it may be good to start with walking or riding a stationary bicycle. Stop if you hurt or feel tired. It's always best to be checked by your doctor before beginning an exercise program.

Physical activity can be structured, as in the form of walking, exercising in a gym, or running, biking, playing soccer, etc., or it can be worked into your daily routine, or both. Once you become fitter and are able to do about an hour a day, you may prefer to break it up into two 30-minute sessions instead of one 60-minute session. That is fine. You may find that you like to do an exercise video in the morning, and then walk the dog at night. Do what works best for you. An ideal fitness routine combines aerobic activity, strength training and stretching. By adding strength training to your workout, you can strengthen your muscles, and increase your lean body mass, which can also help to increase your metabolism and help you lose weight. If you do participate in strength training or weight lifting, it is important to begin with low-resistance exercises, learn good technique and be properly supervised, so that you avoid injury.

Choose an Activity You Enjoy

To begin with, do anything to get moving. The type of physical activity you choose doesn't really matter, as long as it gets you moving and as long as it's safe. The more important part is that you enjoy doing it. Consider whether you're someone who likes to do activities on your own, or whether you would prefer to be with others, in a gym, or on a sports team, for example. You may even be lucky enough to work out with a personal trainer. Being forced to do something you hate day after day won't work for long, so choose something fun. Someone once told me proudly that she had been a member of a gym for three years. She wasn't becoming fitter, though, because she had been to her gym only twice. Clearly, the gym was not a solution for her! On the other hand, some people find it less fun to work out at home, but really enjoy the atmosphere of a gym.

At our center we have a physical activity program for teenagers, run by exercise physiologists. The program is popular with teens because it's fun and they can work out with others their own age. It works well because they are monitored for attendance and progress and receive lots of one-on-one attention.

Once you find something that works for you, it is also good to vary the activity from time to time to prevent boredom, and to challenge new muscles. Read these ideas to get you started:

- Join a dance class, or just put on some music and dance.
- Go for a bike ride outside, or ride a stationary bicycle if you prefer.
- Put an exercise machine, such as a bike, elliptical trainer or treadmill, in front of your television set and watch your favorite TV show while you work out.
- Join a gym, or walk or run on a treadmill, if you have one at home. You can wear a Walkman or iPod and listen to your favorite music while you walk on the treadmill.
- Play tennis, or go golfing with a friend.
- Start swimming.
- Join a school sports team, or start an informal team with some of your friends.
- Do gardening in summer, raking leaves in fall and clearing snow in winter. You will get lots of exercise, and probably earn some money too.
- Ask someone to join you for a walk a few days a week, or take your dog for a walk.
- Consider working out with a friend. Although some people do enjoy exercising alone, many young people tell me they prefer working out or doing activities with someone else. That way, if one is not motivated, the other can encourage him or her to continue.

Yoga

Yoga is a Hindu discipline consisting of a system of exercises to promote spirituality and tranquility, as well as control over mind and body. Yoga's history goes back thousands of years and began in India. Meditation and the various yoga positions make up only a small part of what constitutes the yoga philosophy. Yoga teaches one to rest the mind and find peace and happiness within oneself. It also teaches discipline and concentration.

Yoga provides many potential physical benefits including better posture, strength and flexibility, as well as psychological benefits such as improved mental clarity and decreased stress. Although yoga can be practiced at home, it's best to start by joining a class with an experienced instructor. You should start off slowly, be properly supervised, and should not feel pain during or after completing a class.

Pilates

Pilates, a system of physical exercises, stretching and body conditioning, was originally developed by Joseph Pilates in the 1920s, and is now practiced in studios all over the world. The Pilates method works on strengthening core muscles in the abdominal area and around the spine as well as the muscles surrounding the joints. Its goal is also to improve whole body strength and flexibility.

Organized sports

Although children in the United States tend to become less active as they progress through the teenage years, millions still participate in organized sports. They participate for all sorts of reasons, including the following:

- For social reasons—to make new friends or to spend time with young people with similar interests.
- For health reasons.
- To please others, e.g. their parents.
- For status.
- To gain skills—not only physical skills, but also learning to set goals, cope with success and failure, and work as a team.
- To gain access to financial support, e.g. college scholarships.
- For fun and excitement.

Benefits of organized sports also include improvement of strength, fitness and flexibility, an opportunity to learn life skills such as discipline, feeling a sense of achievement, and improved self-esteem.

Whatever you choose to do, whether it be organized sports, or taking walks with a friend, schedule physical activity into your daily routine, and make it a priority. If you don't plan the time in advance, it won't happen. Go to your calendar now and pencil it in for next week.

Exercise Safely

However you choose to exercise, keep the following safety tips in mind:

- Don't do too much too soon. Allow a few minutes to warm up before exercising and cool down after. Stop exercising if you feel pain.
- Vary your routine to give your body (and muscles) time to recover between workouts. For example, if you run on Mondays and Wednesdays, consider biking or swimming on Tuesdays and Thursdays.
- Wear appropriate, well-fitting shoes, as well as any protective gear recommended for your particular sport.
- Avoid strenuous activity during periods of high heat and humidity. Make sure you remain hydrated by drinking plenty of water.
- Prevent sunburn by using sunscreen with an SPF of at least 15 when exercising outdoors.
- Bicycle accidents are among the leading causes of head injury in children and teenagers. One step that you can take to help prevent head injury is to wear a safety-approved bicycle helmet. It's also important to make sure that your bike (especially its brakes) is in good working order before you head out.
- If you participate in weight training, make sure you learn the correct technique and are properly supervised.
- Don't smoke. Apart from being dangerous to your health, smoking can also result in poor athletic performance.
- Have regular physical check-ups to make sure you are healthy and that there is no contraindication to participation in sports.

Personal Trainers

Some people do best with a personal trainer, who can guide them, motivate them, and hold them accountable for showing up regularly. Many health clubs can provide you with a personal trainer at an additional cost. It is important to keep in mind that not all personal trainers have the same qualifications, and not all are familiar with working with teenagers. Ask about the trainer's certification and experience. Ask if the trainer is certified in CPR (cardiopulmonary resuscitation). Will he or she ask about your health history and keep a record of your progress? Your primary care doctor may be able to provide you with names of certified personal trainers.

Unstructured Physical Activity

Introduce physical activity into your daily routine. With all the energy-saving devices available to us today, one has to make a real effort to get physical activity. We don't routinely take the stairs, walk to a restaurant or the library, wash the dishes by hand, open the garage door or even go to the television set to turn it on. Elevators, drive-through restaurants, dishwashing machines, the Internet, automatic garage door openers and remote controls have taken over. However, making your everyday routine more active is probably as important as doing structured physical activity. Do both! I work on the fourth floor of our building, and I have made a rule that I will not use the elevator. Walking up a few flights of stairs each day makes a difference. Dance, jump, do sit-ups or stretch during television commercials. Help with washing the car or working in the garden. If it's safe and not too far, walk to the store or your friend's home instead of driving. See what you can do to make your day more active. One creative way in which you can measure your activity is by strapping on a pedometer (a device used to record the number of steps you take) and seeing how many steps you take each day. Then challenge yourself to increase that a little each week. Chart the total number of steps you take each day. Aim for about ten thousand steps over the course of a day (equivalent to about five miles). The average person who is not very active takes about two or three thousand a day.

Be Less Inactive

In addition to becoming more active, you also need to become less inactive. Decreasing the amount of time you spend just "sitting around" can have a significant effect on your weight. There are many studies linking obesity to watching too much television. *Yes, those sitcoms and reality shows you watch are probably making you gain weight.* There is evidence that simply by spending less time watching television, one can lose weight. Watching television keeps you from being active, and exposes you to constant snack-food commercials. Advertisers know what they're doing and they know the power they have over us. Sitting in front of that television set makes you a prime target for their commercials. Many people adopt the habit of eating while watching television. When you are engrossed in watching a program, you can easily lose track of what you have eaten. Television keeps you from doing other fun activities and spending time with your friends. The American Academy of Pediatrics recommends limiting media time (including TV) to no more than one to two hours a day. So, why don't you think of all the fun things you could do instead of sitting and staring at that television screen? Meet a friend and go for a walk, play tennis or basketball, start a fun hobby, listen to music and dance, paint a picture or throw a Frisbee. I bet you won't miss that television program at all.

What's Your Excuse?

I have heard every excuse in the book when it comes to having to do physical activity. The most common excuse is that there is no time to exercise. All one needs is at most sixty minutes a day, and if you examine your day, I know you will find the time. Even the president finds time to exercise. If you can't find sixty minutes, cut out some of your television time during the week. If you don't watch TV and still don't find the time during the day, split your workout into two shorter sessions.

Injury is another common complaint that may keep people from exercising. However, in the case of a mild injury, and as long as your doctor agrees, you may still be able to exercise without using the injured part of your body. So, if you hurt your arm, you may still be able to ride a stationary bike, and if you hurt your ankle, you may still be able to use a rowing machine.

Young people may also avoid exercise because they don't belong to a gym and don't own any exercise equipment. Walking or running outside is a great form of exercise. If safety or weather becomes an issue, you can walk up and down the steps in your house, dance to music or jump rope. In bad weather many people even go for walks in shopping malls. You don't need any fancy equipment, a gym membership, or even much time to start becoming fit now. So what's *your* excuse?

Most creative excuses (and solutions)

- "I don't want to get sweaty." Take a shower or a swim afterwards and you'll feel cool and refreshed.
- "I have too much homework to do." Exercise can wake you up and give you an energy boost. You'll probably be more productive after you've done some physical activity.
- "It's too cold to work out." Do something indoors, or if it's not dangerously cold outside, bundle up with layers of clothing and head out anyway. You'll probably warm up very quickly, once you start moving.
- "I am embarrassed to put on gym clothes. I look too fat." You don't have to wear fancy gym clothes. Wear comfortable clothes and good shoes. Once you start working out, you'll feel better about your body too.
- "I have no energy to work out." Regular exercise can increase your energy level. If you continue to feel tired and lack energy, check with your doctor.
- "I don't want to miss my favorite television show." If the show is really important to you, tape it and watch it at a later time. Don't let television control your life.
- "I lost my gym shoes." (I'm serious, I really heard this.) No comment.
- "Our treadmill broke." Don't procrastinate. Make a decision about whether you will have the treadmill fixed soon, buy another one,

or do another form of activity. So many people stop exercising completely because of broken exercise equipment. There are many other options if you want to stay fit.

• "My walking partner has the flu." Send a get-well card, but don't stop being physically active. You could ask one of your parents or another friend to join you for a walk, or put the stationary bicycle in front of the television set and watch your favorite show while you bike.

• "It's boring." Exercise shouldn't be boring. If it is, it means you're probably doing the wrong type of exercise for you. Try something different and vary it from time to time.

• "It's too difficult." You may have pushed yourself too hard. Back off a little. If you have been working out for 30 minutes, try 15 or 20 minutes for a while. If you have been running, perhaps you could alternate walking and running. Exercise should also not hurt. Forget the "no pain, no gain" mentality. If it does hurt, stop or decrease the intensity of your workout until you feel better.

• "I can't exercise for the next few weeks, because we will be traveling." Traveling should not stop you from being active. Wherever you are, you will probably be able to take walks outside, or will have access to a hotel pool or gym. You're all set if you take an active family vacation involving an activity such as hiking, skiing or canoeing, for example.

• "Exercise doesn't work." That's not what studies show. There is lots of evidence to show that exercising regularly is beneficial to your health and can also help you maintain a healthy weight.

• "I'll start tomorrow." Don't put this off until tomorrow. Do something healthy for yourself today. You can start with just a few minutes, and gradually increase the time and intensity of your workout. Do at least some form of activity on a regular basis. Soon you will find that being physically active will become a habit — a good habit.

How to Get Out of a Rut

There may be a time, however, when you lose motivation and it just becomes tough to keep going. Maybe you are not seeing fast results, or maybe you have just become bored with your exercise routine. This is not the time to give up! This is the time, I believe, when we separate those who will succeed from those who will not. Keep going, but change your plan. You may change your workout, or alternate your workouts with another activity. If you have been biking, start jogging, or swimming, or dancing. If you have been exercising alone, ask a friend to join you. Try listening to music. Buy an exercise video. Consider changing the time of day that you exercise. Challenge yourself by setting new goals, and recording them in a journal. Last but not least, enjoy yourself. If you do something you like doing, it will be so much easier to continue. Michael, a sixteen-year-old boy, was exercising for thirty minutes three days a week, and was frustrated because his weight had plateaued. He added two more days of physical activity and within just a few weeks he began seeing and feeling significant results.

11

Modifying Your Behaviors

Changing or modifying your behaviors through various techniques can help you improve your nutrition and increase your physical activity, both of which are key to reaching your goal of permanent weight loss. If you are overweight, you have to make long-term changes with respect to your eating and physical activity in order to lose weight and keep it off. You don't have to change everything at once. Make these healthy changes slowly, one at a time. After a few weeks, the new behavior becomes entrenched, and then you can move on to the next one. This way it won't ever be overwhelming.

Monitor Yourself

One of the most important steps you can take toward reaching your goal to become healthier and lose weight is to monitor yourself. One way in which to do this is by keeping a food-and-activity journal. I discuss this in more detail in chapter 13. When you record all of your intake and activity for a week, you will probably be very surprised, as people tend to underestimate what they eat and overestimate the amount of physical activity they do. The very act of keeping a journal may help you lose weight by making you become more aware of your habits. You can't make changes if you are not aware of what you are doing right now. I heard a funny story at a lecture on weight control. A patient was told that he should record everything he ate in his food journal. It was stressed that nothing, not even drinks, should be left out. He was struggling to recall what he ate at each meal, so he came up with a creative plan. His doctor smiled when he came in the following week with an almost-blank journal and a set of photographs of plates of food. In his journal he had begun to record his meals, but then simply wrote: "see photograph." Although this technique worked for this particular patient, I am not suggesting that you should take pictures of everything you eat. Perhaps you could design your own goal chart, and use stickers for accomplishments. If your goal is to eat five servings of fruits and vegetables each day, check them off one by one, and place a sticker on your chart when you reach five.

Control Your Environment

There are all sorts of triggers in our environment that entice us to do certain things or behave in certain ways. Having a television set in your bedroom will probably increase your chances of watching more TV and being more sedentary. Keeping rich desserts in your house every day will make it more difficult to eat in a healthy way. Having to walk past a donut shop to get to school each day may tempt you to eat donuts. Joining a gym, perhaps together with a friend, makes it more likely that you will do some physical activity because you have paid for your membership.

Try to understand what, other than hunger, triggers you to eat. I have made a list and you can add to it. I have also included an alternate way of dealing with the situation, other than by eating.

- Stress or need for comfort — Some people turn to food when they are stressed and need comfort. Instead of turning to food, you could talk to a family member or friend about your problems.
- Reward — We have been conditioned to associate food with reward. Celebrations and achievements often involve large amounts of food. When you were younger, you may have been rewarded with cookies or sweets if you finished your homework, or if you finished your meal. Instead of considering food as a reward, why don't you reward yourself with a good movie or a good book, or going out with a friend, or even a membership to a local pool or gym?
- Environment — You may find that you always eat more when you visit certain relatives, if you are at a party, or if you are faced with

certain temptations. Plan in advance for these situations and imagine in your mind how you will deal with them. Consider having a healthy snack before you go to the relative's home or the party. In the case of having to walk past a donut shop to get to school, consider taking an alternate route.

- People — You may eat more when you are around certain people. I know of someone who had an aunt who always urged her to eat a little more, or to try some of a second cake too. To her it was a sign of love if you ate her food. If you identify with this situation, don't feel bad about saying no. You could say that the cake looks wonderful, but that you just ate, or that you are trying to avoid sweets. You may have to say no several times at first, but say it in a nice way. Eventually the person will get the message.
- Birthdays and other celebrations — Most of us like to celebrate special occasions with special treats. We have become accustomed to doing so. If we indulge too much or too often, though, it may become a problem. Enjoy some cake or something else that you like at these events, and don't feel bad about it. Instead of automatically going back for seconds, eat slowly and then decide whether you really want that second piece. You could also balance out the day by eating healthily at the other meals. Don't be tempted to skip meals because of a party. You will only set yourself up for trouble (such as bingeing) later on.
- Depression — Some people turn to food when they feel depressed or lonely. If this happens to you on a regular basis, speak to a parent and your doctor to see about other ways to manage your depression.
- Boredom — I have had so many teenagers tell me they eat when they are bored. Do you? You can avoid boredom by structuring your day in advance. Visualize the day in your mind for a few moments. Decide when you will do any homework or projects. If you know you have free time, you can plan to meet a friend. Start a hobby, which you can pick up whenever you have unstructured time. If you know you are not hungry and are still tempted to eat, delay the urge by taking a five or ten minute walk first. The urge might pass and you will have done something good for yourself.

• The food is there — Some people are tempted to eat when they simply see certain foods. Do you find that when you have a carton of ice cream in the freezer, it beckons you to eat it? Or how about a chocolate cake on the kitchen counter, or an open bag of chips in the pantry? Perhaps there are times when you're not hungry, but you feel compelled to eat if you're faced with a table full of food at a party or buffet. If those situations tempt you, you are not alone. Don't set yourself up for failure by regularly having temptations around. Ask everyone at home if they will support you in this attempt. Have lots of healthy foods such as fruits and vegetables and low-fat yogurts that you can snack on when you're hungry. Put less-healthy foods at the back of the fridge or pantry, so you are less likely to reach for them. Buy snacks in single-serving sizes instead of large bags, so that you will be less likely to eat more than you really need.

See if any of the above situations trigger you to eat. If they do, think about whether you could deal with those situations in another way. I also want to challenge you to spend some time thinking about your environment in general and to come up with ways in which you can make it more health-friendly for you.

We're Too Busy

I believe that one of the biggest problems contributing to weight gain is our hectic schedules. Many families in my clinic tell me they have no time to have dinner together. They don't have the time to sit down to eat, let alone plan and shop for healthy meals. Many of the decisions we make regarding our health are made on the spur of the moment. We may or may not exercise depending on whether or not we find the time on a particular day. We help ourselves to what happens to be in the fridge, or if we have not had lunch, we will pick up something from a fast-food store, or even a vending machine. This will not work. We can't "wing it" this way. In the twenty-first century, active planning is necessary to stay healthy and to avoid piling on the pounds. Today, unfortunately, the natural tendency for many people seems to be to gain too much weight, unless they make a concerted effort not to.

So, make health a priority. Schedule at least thirty to sixty minutes of activity into your day. Take a walk with a family member or friend, or ask your parents if you can join a health club together. Ask your family to shop so that you always have nutritious foods in the fridge. Include meats and fish, fresh and dried fruits, plain popcorn and high-fiber cereals. Other good choices are whole-grain breads, and low-fat dairy products such as milk, yogurt and frozen yogurt. Ask them to clear out the white-flour products, sugary cereals, chips and sodas. Why don't you start by doing that right now? Whenever possible, decide in advance where you will eat your meals on a particular day. If you're going out and know there won't be much time to stop for lunch, take along a sandwich and a fruit. There are also many other ways in which you could modify your environment. For example, if your parents routinely pick you up from school, you could ask them to pick you up ten minutes later. During those ten minutes you could walk around the school track a few times. You've got to "grab" those few minutes when you can. One mother of a young boy who was inactive and very overweight made the excuse that her son had no time to exercise. All I could think was that he had no time *not* to.

An Apple a Day?

Joan was the new receptionist for a lawyer in a prestigious law firm. She shared a desk with Stacy, the meticulously neat secretary of that lawyer's partner. Joan had tried for years to lose weight and had all but given up. Her life was hurried and she felt she had no time to exercise. She hardly had time to cook, and at her previous job had developed the habit of snacking at her desk when she found the time. Stacy did not like a messy environment, and could not tolerate crumbs on her desk. Because she had been there longer, she made the rule that no food other than apples could be eaten at their desk. Joan protested that she didn't eat apples, but quickly changed her mind when she bit into the juicy red apple that Stacy handed her.

From then on, an apple it was. Eight weeks later, Joan stood in front of Stacy and said: "Look what you did to me!" Before Stacy could become concerned, Joan added, "I've lost ten pounds since I have been here. I have never been able to do that before." Simply modifying Joan's environment by not allowing snacking at her desk allowed her to lose the weight.

Change Your Attitude/Beliefs

Constant negative thinking can stand in the way of reaching your goals. Banish thoughts like: "I'll never lose weight" or "I always fail." Replace them with "I'm doing something good for myself now" and "I won't give up because I know I can succeed." You must change your negative thinking into believing that you can achieve what you set out to accomplish. It is also important, of course, that you set realistic goals and have realistic expectations.

Respect yourself

Like yourself for who you are now, not for someone you will become when you lose weight. Losing weight will not change the person you are inside. Recently I was so upset when I saw a "reality" TV show that drastically transformed women's appearances. After one woman's transformation was complete, she was told in effect that she had now changed into a wonderful person. Diet, exercise and plastic surgery, although they can change appearances, can't make a good person. Begin to feel good about yourself now, and you will find it easier to treat yourself well and to reach your goal. One young girl had such dislike for herself that as soon as she started losing weight she regained the weight, because she felt that she was not deserving of a better life. Don't do that to yourself. Have respect for yourself and for your body.

Reward yourself

Feeling stronger, fitter and more energized is already a significant reward. As you start losing weight by eating healthily and by being more active, you will probably become even more motivated. Set both short-term and long-term goals and reward yourself as you reach each goal. For example, your long-term goal may be to become fitter and to lose a total of ten pounds. You can break this up into smaller goals by aiming to lose two or three pounds per month for four months and then working on maintaining that weight. As you reach each goal you could reward yourself in a small way, perhaps with a CD or tickets to a concert. Most often, though, reaching your goal will be rewarding enough.

Learn how to cope with stress

Many people gain excessive weight by eating for emotional reasons rather than for hunger reasons. They cope with sadness, loneliness or stressful situations by eating, rather than by dealing with them in other, healthier ways. Does this sound familiar? If it does, don't wait. Talk to your healthcare provider who can help you with recommendations to manage stress. Some forms of stress can be relieved by exercise and relaxation techniques. More severe stress, anxiety and depression can be helped by therapy, and medication if needed.

Lighten Up!

Learn to prioritize and give time and thought to the things that really matter. Remember to make time for fun! Don't use up all your energy worrying about the unimportant things in life.

Let's Summarize Your Treatment Plan

Remember these ten key principles:

1. Make a commitment
   You must make a commitment to become healthier and fitter.
2. Become motivated
   Find out what motivates you. Does health motivate you, and the fact that you don't want to develop diabetes or heart disease? Are you motivated because you want to have more stamina to be able to participate in sports? Do you want to lose weight because you

feel it may improve your social life, or because you want to be able to buy clothes that fit? You are much more likely to be successful if you are motivated to change.

3. Write down your goals
   Make clear goals—both short-term and long-term. Write them down, and revise them from time to time. You're unlikely to reach your goals when you don't know what they are.

4. Have a sensible nutrition plan
   Eat regular balanced meals and pay attention to portion sizes. Forget about fad diets and save yourself a lot of time, money and aggravation. Start your sensible eating plan today and be one step closer to becoming healthier and fitter.
   - Favor complex carbohydrates over simple carbohydrates.
   - Try to get about three servings of low-fat or non-fat dairy products daily.
   - Limit your intake of total and saturated fat.
   - Get lots of fiber in your diet by eating whole grains (instead of refined grains) and at least five servings of fruits and vegetables every day.
   - Drink water and non-fat milk instead of juices and sodas.

5. Be more active
   Aim to get about an hour of physical activity on most days of the week. Start slowly and gradually increase the time and intensity as you are able. Don't do too much too soon. Remember that any amount of physical activity is better than none at all. Add little bits of activity into your daily routine too.

6. Be less inactive
   Limit your "media time" (including television) to no more than one to two hours daily, and aim for less than that. Instead of feeling deprived, think of all the fun things you could do instead.

7. Take small positive steps
   Aim for gradual change. Taking small steps in the right direction can lead to great results, and you'll never feel overwhelmed. Make tiny lasting changes that become habits, and then move on to the next one. Examples are switching from white rice to brown rice, or from whole milk to 1 percent milk, or cutting out sodas.

8. Change your attitude
   - Have a positive attitude and believe that you can succeed.
   - Instead of thinking of a short-term plan with rapid weight loss, think of a long-term plan and a permanent healthy weight. Don't let minor set-backs discourage you. They're normal. Keep going.
   - Like yourself for who you are now and not for who you will become.
   - Treat your body and yourself with respect.
9. Change your behaviors
   - Avoid situations that trigger your overeating, such as all-you-can eat buffets, for example. If you can't avoid them, plan for them in advance.
   - Change your environment to promote more physical activity. For example, if you can't join a gym, you could invest in an exercise bicycle or a treadmill.
   - Change the way you relate to food and your environment. If you always turn to food when stressed, find healthier ways to cope with your stress.
   - Do not be afraid to ask for help if you are depressed, too stressed, engage in binge eating, or things don't go as well as planned.
10. Reward yourself
   Give yourself little rewards as you reach your goals. Although feeling healthier and being fitter is its own reward, there is nothing wrong with buying yourself something you've wanted, within reason. These rewards are extra little bonuses that may help to motivate you.

   Keep a list of these principles handy and refer to them from time to time. If things are not progressing as they should, go over the principles and make sure you are following each one.

12

Medical Treatments for the Overweight

Medical problems can cause weight gain (rarely) or can result from being overweight. It's important for you to follow up with your physician as recommended. Your doctor can check your weight, assess whether you are healthy, and evaluate lab tests if necessary. He or she can also answer any questions you may have about your health, and help you establish ongoing goals. If you have developed any medical complications related to weight gain, including such problems as diabetes, high blood pressure, joint problems, hormonal problems or elevated cholesterol levels, it will be important to follow up on a regular basis. Weight loss and physical activity will be a key part of treatment. Sometimes medications will be recommended in addition to lifestyle changes.

Psychotherapy

Some people who are overweight have an eating disorder, namely binge-eating disorder, or they may have psychological problems such as anxiety or depression. It is important to address these problems in addition to making nutritional changes. Their treatment will usually include some form of psychotherapy. This may take the form of individual, family, or group therapy.

Individual therapy such as cognitive behavioral therapy can lead to better understanding of one's behaviors and to identifying alternative healthier behaviors. For example, if you always turn to food when you are stressed, you can learn other healthier ways to deal with your stress.

If you are a younger teenager struggling with weight problems, family therapy may be more helpful, as it would be best to address any problems you may have in the context of your family and home environment. You will find it easier to reach your goals if your family is supportive of them. Family therapy provides a chance to constructively address family conflicts that contribute to eating problems.

Group therapy may be another option for you. Within the group you can address your concerns in a safe environment, and find support from others with similar problems. It is often less expensive, too.

Medication for Psychiatric Problems

Some people who are overweight (as well as some who are not overweight) have problems such as depression or anxiety disorders. These problems may contribute to weight gain. Besides offering psychotherapy, psychiatrists can prescribe medications to treat these conditions.

Medication to Treat Obesity

A number of medications have been and are being tested for the treatment of obesity. So far, none of these medications has completely lived up to our expectations, and they all have side effects. While most side effects of these prescription medications are mild, serious side effects have been reported. Not long ago, a combination of medications known as "phen-phen" was taken off the market because it was found to increase the risk of heart disease. For this reason, among others, weight-loss medication should be used only for patients at increased medical risk because of their obesity, not for those who want to lose a few pounds to look better.

Two of the medications that are currently approved for the treatment of obesity are Orlistat and Sibutramine.

In December 2003, Orlistat (Xenical), which has been used as a treatment for obesity in adults, was approved by the Food and Drug Administration (FDA) for the management of obesity in teenagers aged 12 to 16 years. This medication works locally in the gut by decreasing the absorption of fat from the diet by about 30 percent. Because the medication also decreases the absorption of some vitamins, a daily multivitamin should be taken.

Sibutramine (Meridia) suppresses appetite by altering chemicals in the brain. Safety and effectiveness of this medication have not been established in pediatric patients.

Each patient responds differently to these medications, but they usually lead to only modest amounts of weight loss. Weight-loss medications are not the magic answer, and should never replace healthy lifestyle behaviors such as healthy eating and regular physical activity. In some situations, though, they can help people maintain a healthier routine. The research will be ongoing to try to develop more effective medications.

Surgery

An in-depth discussion of various surgical techniques is outside the scope of this book. Surgery is a last resort in the treatment of obesity in young people. You will probably read a lot about gastric bypass surgery. Gastric bypass works by altering the size and shape of the stomach and small intestine so that the body can absorb only small amounts of food. There are many risks involved with surgery and people considering this type of procedure should have extensive counseling before undergoing the surgery.

13

Maintaining a Healthy Lifestyle

Losing the weight is only the first step on the way to a new, healthier life. You have to keep the weight off over the long term.

Josh's Story

Fourteen-year-old Josh lost 25 pounds and has maintained a healthy weight for over a year now. He also has a great attitude. He has become used to fellow students asking him how he manages to keep his weight down, and he enjoys sharing his story. "I never skip meals, but now I have one plate of food instead of two, and one bowl of cereal instead of two. I used to reach automatically for a second serving, but now I stop to ask myself if I'm still hungry. If I am, I'll have that second helping, but usually the answer is no. So I save those calories for when I really want something. I don't snack mindlessly anymore, but I do still eat sweets sometimes. I'll have cake at a birthday party, and I eat frozen yogurt quite often. I try to eat the fat-free or low-fat kind." Because we know that people who exercise regularly are more likely to maintain healthy weights, I asked Josh whether he participated in any physical activity. Josh answered: "Working out has become a part of my life and I love it. Now if I don't do some type of physical activity every day, I really miss it. I ride a bike or play basketball outside or just go for a walk. My gym teacher at school is amazed at how fit I have become. Last year, when we did the mile run, I finished up near the end, and this year I finished second. Maybe I'll be first next year! You've got to have goals."

A Reality Check

I don't want to be negative at this point in the book, but I do want to be realistic. You know that it's not easy to lose weight, but it may be even more difficult keeping the weight off. Many people who lose weight regain the weight they lost. Sometimes this pattern is repeated several times. This is more likely to happen if you go on restrictive or fad diets. These are the "yo-yo" dieters. You've probably heard of them and perhaps you were one of them. The aim of this book is to help you reach a healthy weight range in a safe way, and maintain it forever. You can do it with some planning. The important thing is to continue a healthy way of eating and exercising even after you have reached your goal. Many people, once they reach their target weight, relax and return to their old lifestyles. Don't fall into this trap, because you will be back where you started. So, when you reach your goal weight, follow the steps below to make sure that you stay in control.

Review Your Goals

Have you reached your goal weight or do you still need to lose more weight? Remember that your goal weight is not a single number – rather it is a range. It's normal for your weight to fluctuate by a few pounds. If you are unsure of your healthy weight range, check with your doctor. Review your other goals too. You may have reached your desired weight, but may want to become fitter to participate in a certain sports event, for example. Continually setting goals and challenging yourself can help keep you motivated.

Monitor Yourself

Although it is a good idea to have an assessment (and, if necessary, treatment) by your healthcare provider, it is also important for you to develop skills so that you can continue to monitor yourself forever. For example, let us say you went to your doctor and together you set a goal for you to lose 15 pounds. You enlisted the help of a dietitian with whom you met every two weeks for five months. You kept track of what you were eating and how much you were exercising, and you lost the 15 pounds. What then? Without continuing to keep some record of what you do, it becomes more difficult to stay on track. The good news is that with a little effort, and self-monitoring, you can maintain a healthy lifestyle and a healthy weight.

There are two simple ways of monitoring yourself at home. One is by recording your physical activity and what you eat in a journal, and the other is by weighing yourself regularly. There is no need to become obsessive about what you eat or how much you weigh. On the other hand, monitoring your progress by weighing yourself weekly and by journaling can be a strong motivator, and can help to keep you on the right path.

Keep a food and activity journal

You may use any journal or notebook to write down everything you eat and drink, as well as the type and amount of physical activity you do. Make a point of recording in your journal at least every evening. For journaling to be effective, you must write down everything (except water perhaps), and you may not be accurate if you wait until the following day. People often tend to underestimate what they eat. Journals can be very helpful for several reasons: they can make you more aware of what and when you eat, and they enable you to monitor your progress. If you wish to do so, you can take these logs to your physician and dietitian so that they can evaluate your eating and physical activity habits.

At the end of the chapter, I have included sample journal logs. Feel free to fill them in to get started.

Weigh yourself

Weighing yourself weekly can help you keep track of your progress and can also be motivating. It's usually not necessary to weigh yourself more often. I have heard of people weighing themselves several times a day. This can contribute to obsessiveness, and will not give you any useful information about your weight status. Once a day is not extreme as long as you don't expect to see changes daily. I recommend that you weigh yourself once a week, in the morning, before breakfast. Record your weekly weights in your journal.

Note: If you have or have had an eating disorder, you may sometimes be advised not to weigh yourself at home.

Maintain a Healthy Eating Plan

Are you satisfied with the way you are eating? Are there any changes you should make? Review below:

Shop for healthy foods

This applies to everyone who does the food shopping for your home. Make a list before you go to the store and stick to your list. Spend most of your time along the perimeter of the store where you will find the fresh fruits and vegetables, meats, fish and dairy products. Don't spend as much time in the center of the store with the snack foods. Don't be fooled by nutrition labels with words such as reduced-fat, fat-free and light. Many reduced-fat and fat-free items are packed with calories. Don't shop when you're hungry and don't buy food you don't want to eat.

Make healthy choices at home and in restaurants...

There is no perfect "diet," but remember to keep some basic principles in mind when you cook and when you go out to eat. When cooking at home, bake, grill or "oven-fry" foods rather than frying or pan-frying them. Remove the skin from chicken before cooking it and cut all visible fats off meat. If you don't cook, ask your Mom or Dad if they will do this for the family. These are basic healthy principles that can apply to almost anyone. Make sure that you get enough calcium in your diet, and use low-fat (or non-fat) milk products when possible. Fill up on colorful salads, but be cautious about creamy salad dressings, which can add hundreds of calories. A little olive oil and balsamic vinegar is a better choice than a Caesar dressing. When cooking eggs, use fewer yolks.

When eating out, ask to have the sauces and dressings served on the side, and if portions are too large, put some food on the side to share or take home. Studies show that, in general, people eat more calories and fewer fruits and vegetables when eating outside of the home. On the other hand, eating out does not need to destroy your healthy routine. With a little planning, you will be able to have a healthy meal in almost any restaurant. To make it easier for you, choose restaurants that offer healthy, tasty foods, and order your food as you would like to have it prepared. Many people take in hundreds of calories before they are even served their meal by eating several slices of bread or munching on chips. If you are going to eat bread, eat only one slice, or eat it when your meal is served. If you decide to order meat or fish, most restaurants will prepare it grilled or baked, even if that is not indicated on the menu. Recently I went to a restaurant and ordered a grilled chicken sandwich and a salad. I asked them to hold the fries and the mayonnaise and butter on the roll, and to serve a vinaigrette dressing instead of the creamy ranch dressing. I still had a wonderful meal and the waitress did not look too upset. I figured out that I saved at least five hundred calories at that meal.

...and at parties

There is no reason not to have a good time at parties just because you are watching your weight. Eat something light before you go to the party so that you won't be as tempted by all the snack food. Don't skip meals. If you think you may eat more at an evening party, make sure you eat a healthy breakfast and lunch. At a buffet, choose the food items you really like, eat slowly, and don't go back for seconds.

Traveling

You can still have all the fun without having to give up your healthy routine when you travel. I often hear the excuse that people couldn't eat healthily or be active because they were on vacation. In fact, although vacations do disrupt normal schedules, they often provide many opportunities to try new activities and even new foods that taste good and are good for you.

If you travel with your parents, ask them to help you by planning fun activities together. Depending on where you vacation, you could go hiking, swimming, biking or canoeing with the family. If these are not possibilities, ask your parents to join you for a daily sightseeing trip by foot. Walking provides a great opportunity to really get to know your surroundings. Also, many hotels and resorts have health clubs and indoor pools, so bad weather should not ruin your plans to be active.

Stick to a few basic rules and you will be able to maintain a reasonably healthy eating plan while away from home. Stick to your regular routine as closely as possible. Eat regular meals, and include breakfast even if you wake up late. A good breakfast will give you energy and help prevent overeating later in the day. Allow yourself some special treats while traveling, but make up for this by eating more nutritious foods when you can. Make a point of eating lots of fruits and vegetables each day. You can do this even on vacation! If you're staying in a hotel or apartment, keep fresh fruits and other healthy snacks on hand so that you won't be tempted to eat "whatever's available" when hunger strikes. When eating out at restaurants, ask for grilled, broiled or baked entrees instead of fried, and request sauces on the side.

Flying

If you're flying to your destination, it's worth planning ahead. Today airlines rarely serve meals on domestic flights, so you may be tempted to eat less-nutritious food (such as fast foods, chips or candy bars) bought in the airport. Instead, plan ahead by packing healthy snacks such as a whole-wheat sandwich and fruit, or low-fat trail mix, or allow yourself time to sit down at a restaurant and have a good meal. While waiting for your flight, use the opportunity to walk around, because once in the air, you'll be sitting for a long time.

The Beach

Beach vacations bring to mind thoughts of sand, seagulls and surfing, as well as pizza, boardwalk fries and ice-cream cones. Don't panic. If you're traveling with your parents, ask them to shop for some basic foods at the nearby supermarket. Buy cereal and milk (if you have a fridge), whole-wheat bread for sandwiches, and lots of fresh fruits. If you have a craving for something like ice cream, make it a low-fat frozen yogurt, and if you want to have pizza, go ahead, but make it one slice instead of two, and then fill up on healthier choices. When driving to the beach you may find very few restaurants other than fast-food restaurants. If you don't find a place with healthier options, customize your order. For example, order the burger without the cheese and mayonnaise, and order a side salad instead of fries. Pack lots of healthy foods such as rice cakes, dried fruit and carrots to snack on if you're still hungry. Carry bottled water with you to drink instead of sodas.

Cruising

Going on a cruise vacation can be a challenge if you're trying to eat healthily. Long unstructured days, all-you-can-eat buffets, midnight feasts and free ice-cream bars are hard to resist. However, even on a cruise you can stay in control. Most cruises now offer healthier menu choices. Some even make the nutritional content of the foods available right on the menu, so you know what you're ordering. Enjoy your favorites at the buffet, but have one serving instead of two and balance higher-calorie, higher-fat choices with more nutritious ones so you don't overdo it.

You'll have plenty of opportunity to be active on a cruise ship. Most ships have at least one health club, a swimming pool and a walking deck, and offer games such as basketball and table tennis. Take advantage of time spent on land by walking instead of driving, and participating in fun activities such as snorkeling. Happy sailing!

Practice Good Eating Habits

You can practice eating slowly by chewing your food well and putting your fork or spoon down after each mouthful. Eating slowly will allow time for your body to realize that your stomach is full, and you will probably enjoy your food more and may eat fewer calories. We are so hurried these days that we often finish a meal in only a few minutes. In Europe, where a smaller percentage of adults are overweight, people eat more leisurely meals even though they eat smaller portions. And they enjoy their meals!

Continue to be conscious about what you eat. I know of someone who never ordered dessert, but took tastes of everyone else's dessert. She convinced herself that little tastes here and there did not count. As you know, that's not so. Grabbing a handful of chips or licking the icing bowl or finishing someone else's cake all adds up. It's fine to do once in a while, but be aware that you are doing so by writing it down in your food journal. Eat mindfully. That means that you should pay attention to your eating, rather than eating while you are doing something else. Designate an eating place in your home, like the dining room table or the kitchen table. Don't eat while watching television and don't eat in your bedroom. And, although many of us may have been guilty of this sin, don't eat in the car! (It's dangerous, too.)

Snack on Healthy Foods, but Don't Deny Yourself an Occasional Treat

Keep healthy snacks easily accessible. This way you are more likely to reach for them when hunger strikes. Your fridge at home should be filled with items such as fresh fruits and vegetables, skim or low-fat milk products, and lean cuts of meat such as turkey breast. Your pantry should be stocked with dried fruits, raisins, peanut butter and almonds, rice cakes, dried popcorn kernels for air popping and high fiber cereals, and your freezer could hold frozen vegetables, frozen berries for shakes, and low-fat frozen yogurt. Have whole-grain bread available for sandwiches. Prepare a bowl of cut-up vegetables to eat with a low-fat dip. If you have a craving for a certain food, it's okay to indulge, as long as it's only once in a while. Don't deny yourself. It will make it easier for you knowing that you can occasionally have that special treat without feeling guilty.

Find Ways to Distract Yourself

How about making a list of a few alternative activities to do when tempted to eat outside of regular meals and snacks? I'll start the list and you add to it.

1. Take a five-minute walk.
2. Call a friend.
3. Do something creative, such as drawing, or write a poem or a song.
4. Do a few stretching exercises.
5. Take a bath while you listen to music.
6. Drink a cup of herbal tea.
7. Write a letter to a friend you haven't seen in a while. These days, it's such a surprise to receive a letter instead of e-mail.
8. Dance to your favorite music or music video.
9. Take deep breaths and relax for a few minutes.

10, 11, 12 ... the rest are up to you!

Continue to Be Physically Active

Now that you are in your maintenance phase, are you satisfied with the amount of physical activity you are doing, or do you find that you are spending more time watching television? Remember that if you continue to participate in some form of physical activity, you have a much better chance of keeping the weight off. Be physically active for about an hour on most days of the week. For some of you this may mean running or biking. For others, an hour's walk is fine. Do what you feel comfortable doing, as long as you are moving. Add interest to your routine by varying it, and by continually challenging yourself.

Add Bits of Activity Into Your Daily Routine

Plan to walk to the store instead of driving, or to use the stairs instead of the elevator. With friends, go bowling or ice-skating instead of going to the movies. I found it funny when someone once gave me a ride to the health club and she drove around for five minutes to find a parking spot near the door. She was going to walk on the treadmill for one hour, but she didn't want to walk the extra few steps from the car to the door!

Get Enough Sleep

This sounds contradictory, doesn't it? Well it's not. People who don't get enough sleep and who are overtired can't take care of themselves as well and often don't eat as well as they should. Being overtired and stressed can also lead to overeating, an irritable mood, and will make it harder for you to adhere to a physical activity schedule. You don't want to be falling asleep on the treadmill, do you? Make sure that you get enough sleep at night so that you will have more energy and will find it easier maintaining your healthy lifestyle.

Angela's story

Angela, an eighteen-year-old student, found it difficult to keep her weight down although she said she had tried everything. When she told me her schedule, I wasn't surprised that she had struggled. Angela stayed up till past midnight almost every night, doing homework or checking her e-mail. When she woke up in the morning she was so tired that she couldn't eat breakfast. At school she had a small lunch in the cafeteria or from the vending machine. By mid-afternoon, when she returned home, she was starving and ate almost anything she could find in the fridge. Many evenings she kept on eating until she felt sick, and then, too uncomfortable to go to bed, she would stay up and work late. So the cycle would repeat itself. Because of her exhaustion, she didn't do much physical activity.

When I challenged her to go to bed earlier, she declined, saying that she would never be able to complete her work. Reluctantly, she eventually agreed to try a new routine for a week only. She began on a Sunday night, put her books away and went to bed at 10:30. She set her alarm for 6:45 and made herself eat a small bowl of cereal with half a banana. It wasn't easy because Angela wasn't used to eating breakfast, and she was convinced on that first day that she wasn't going to keep this up. Still, she had a good lunch at school that day, and when she came home and went straight to the fridge as usual, she found that she wasn't quite as hungry as she used to be. She had a sandwich, and a large bowl of frozen yogurt, but stopped at that, and then because she didn't feel as uncomfortable as she usually did, she was able to concentrate on her homework. To her surprise, by early evening she had completed it all, and still had time to spare. Because Angela had made the commitment to me, she resisted the temptation to stay up too late, and again switched her light off at 10:30. The next morning was a little easier, and Angela noticed that she felt less irritable. Everyone at home noticed the difference too, and they all tried to be supportive. Her mother cooked "extra special" dinners, and the family tried to make an effort to sit down to dinners together. By the end of the week, Angela was eating a good dinner at 7:00 P.M. and found that she was actually looking forward to eating breakfast. Because she was getting enough sleep, she had more energy and committed to adding an evening walk to her routine.

Don't Give Up

Don't give in to set-backs. Everyone has them. Expect your weight to fluctuate a little. If your weight increases, start recording in your food journal more diligently, or increase your activity a little. If you don't exercise for a day or two, or you eat too much dessert on one day, don't be too hard on yourself. Keep trying! The key is to get back on track as soon as possible. That may be the difference between failure and success.

Follow Up as Needed

Make sure to follow up with your primary-care physician or other health care providers if needed. Together you should also make a plan to deal with setbacks if they occur.

Work on Your Self-esteem

Even though almost 65 percent of adults in the United States are overweight or obese, there is still stigmatization of overweight people in this country. This should not be acceptable. Dealing with this on a day-to-day basis can lead to feelings of shame, and can result in low self-esteem and even isolation. Once you start becoming more active and eating more healthfully, you will feel more motivated and your self-esteem will begin to improve. However, you should not have to wait to feel good about yourself. It is easier to take care of yourself and do good things for your body if you have respect for it, than if you loathe it. So, replace negative thoughts with positive ones. Stop criticizing yourself and think about your good attributes. Decide to continue to eat healthily and to remain active, not because you need to change the way you look, but rather because you want to be healthier, fitter, and have more energy.

Get Support

Maintaining a healthy lifestyle is much easier if you have the support of your family and friends. Get support by surrounding yourself with people who have your best interests at heart. Avoid people who are negative about your goals and successes or who try to undermine your efforts. It's a sad fact that not all friends share in one's motivation to lose weight. For some, it's just not a priority, while others may fear losing the buddy they can hang out with to eat and watch television. It is also not unusual for friends to be jealous of another's weight loss. On the other hand, with them on board, you have an advantage. You can plan active get-togethers and weekends. If you go out to eat, you can choose restaurants that offer healthier choices, and you are less likely to be sabotaged in your attempts to be healthy.

Remember the Basics

If you get off track, remember your ABC's to help you get back on track:

A — Activity: Do some form of physical activity on most days.
B — Breakfast: Eat breakfast every morning.
C — Calcium: Make sure you get enough calcium in your diet. This can be in the form of low-fat (or non-fat) dairy products.

D — Drink plenty of water.

E — Eat regularly to avoid excessive hunger and cravings. Don't skip meals.

F — Fiber: Get enough fiber in your diet by eating whole grains and at least five servings of fruits and vegetables a day.

G — Set goals for yourself

Daily Log

Date:
Breakfast:

Lunch:

Snack:

Dinner:

No. of 8-oz. cups/glasses of water: _____
No. of servings of fruits/vegetables (aim for at least 5 total): _____
Physical activity: _____ minutes
TV/computer/video games (total time spent): _____
Additional notes:

Weekly Log—End of Week 1 (2, 3, etc.)

Date:
Weight:
Total hours of physical activity:
Total TV/computer/video games hours spent:
Goals for next week:

Continue your journal on your own or with the help of your healthcare provider or parents.

14

Eating Disorders

I felt that it was important to include a chapter on eating disorders in a book that deals with weight concerns in teenagers. First of all, eating disorders usually begin in the teenage years. Secondly, you need to know that if you go on an overly restrictive diet, you may put yourself at risk for developing an eating disorder, in addition to other health problems. Also, although most do not, some people who are overweight do have an eating disorder — binge-eating disorder.

What Are Eating Disorders?

Eating disorders are serious medical illnesses that can have extremely harmful health consequences. People who suffer from eating disorders have disturbances in eating habits, excessive concerns about body weight and shape, and low self-esteem. Eating disorders affect not only every aspect of the individual's life, but also the lives of the people close to them. About eight million people in the United States suffer from eating disorders. Eating disorders usually begin in the teenage years, but they can affect people of all age groups. Some people still think eating disorders affect only females, but that is not true. At least 10 percent of people with eating disorders are male.

The best-known eating disorders are anorexia nervosa and bulimia nervosa, but there are many others that are not formally defined which are just as serious. These eating disorders fall under the category "eating disorders not otherwise specified" or "EDNOS," and this category includes binge-eating disorder. Below I have listed the key features of anorexia nervosa, bulimia and binge-eating disorder.

Anorexia nervosa

Anorexia nervosa is a serious, potentially life-threatening illness in which patients literally starve themselves in order to become thinner and thinner. They have an intense fear of gaining weight or becoming fat. Symptoms of anorexia nervosa include the following:

- Excessive weight loss/refusing to maintain at least a minimally normal weight for age and height, due to restriction of calorie intake.
- Intense fear of gaining weight.
- Disturbance in body image.
- In women who have begun menstruating, the absence of at least three consecutive menstrual periods.

Note: Some people with anorexia nervosa may engage in binge eating or purging (self-induced vomiting, or abuse of pills such as laxatives or diuretics).

Anorexia nervosa often begins with a diet, but instead of coming off the diet when a healthy weight is reached, patients with anorexia continue to diet and set lower and lower weight goals.

Bulimia nervosa

Bulimia is a serious eating disorder that affects about 1 to 2 percent of teenage girls and young adult women. Many more young women, especially those in college, may have milder forms of the illness. About 10 percent of people with bulimia are male.

Patients with bulimia:

- Engage in recurrent episodes of binge eating — eating excessive amounts of food in a relatively short period of time, with a sense of lack of control over the eating behavior.
- Engage in recurrent behaviors to try to rid themselves of the extra calories from bingeing — self-induced vomiting, abuse of laxatives, diuretics or other medications, fasting, or excessive exercising.
- Place a high value on their body weight and shape, which strongly influences the way they feel about themselves. They are usually of normal weight or they may be slightly overweight.

In order to make the diagnosis of bulimia, the person must have engaged in the binge eating and compensatory behaviors, on average, at least twice a week for three months.

Note: It is important for you to know that these behaviors are harmful and can lead to serious complications, including heart rhythm disturbances and even death. Unfortunately, patients with bulimia can go undiagnosed for a long time because they may hide their illness, feeling ashamed and disgusted about their behaviors.

Binge-eating disorder (BED)

Binge-eating disorder, like bulimia, is a serious illness, in which patients have recurrent episodes of binge eating. It differs from bulimia in that there are no recurrent compensatory behaviors to control weight, although there may be attempts at dieting. Binge-eating disorder affects between 2 and 5 percent of Americans and occurs in both males and females (females more often than males and adults more often than teenagers). Up to 30 percent of patients seen at weight-loss clinics for the treatment of obesity suffer from binge-eating disorder. Low self-esteem, a parent with depression, exposure to teasing about weight, and restrictive dieting may all put one at risk for BED. To make the diagnosis of binge-eating disorder, the binge eating must occur, on average, at least two days a week for six months. Patients with binge-eating disorder are usually, but not always, overweight. (Binge-eating disorder is treated more fully in chapter 3.)

What Causes Eating Disorders?

There is no single cause for eating disorders. Instead, there are often several factors that play a part in determining whether someone will develop an eating disorder. These include our culture and the media, personal and family factors, and genetics, among other causes.

Culture and the media

Our culture and the media have a strong influence on children and teenagers. Although eating disorders occur in all cultures, they are more common in developed countries and Western cultures that place a high value on appearance, and promote extreme thinness in women and muscularity in men. Young people at risk, who are constantly exposed to media images of very thin women and extremely muscular men, may be at increased risk for the development of an eating disorder or at least body-image dissatisfaction.

Personality and personal factors

Most people who develop eating disorders have low self-esteem. Also, individuals with depression or anxiety disorders may be at increased risk for the development of an eating disorder. People with certain personalities tend to be more at risk for certain types of eating disorders. For example, those who develop anorexia nervosa tend to be more perfectionistic, introverted, and eager to please and want to avoid conflict, while those with bulimia are more extroverted, dramatic and impulsive. People with binge-eating disorder often have a history of being exposed to negative comments about their weight. Of course this is not always the case.

Families

Not everyone who develops an eating disorder comes from a troubled family. However, someone who has a family that has great difficulty communicating or dealing with conflict, or in which there has been a separation, may be at increased risk. Sometimes stress in the family results from the eating disorder, rather than being a cause of it.

Genetics

Although a lot more research is needed, it seems, from family studies, as if genetics plays an important role in determining whether or not a person is predisposed to developing an eating disorder. Eating disorders tend to run in families. Not everyone who is exposed to our culture with its high value placed on thinness will develop an eating disorder. This has led to the belief that certain people are genetically at higher risk.

Friends

Having friends who engage in dieting or eating disordered behavior can increase one's risk.

Illness and other stress

Chronic illnesses such as diabetes mellitus, as well as stressful life events such as leaving home for college, may trigger an eating disorder.

Athletics

Certain athletic activities requiring a low body weight (such as ballet, track and gymnastics) can set one up for over-exercising and eating disorders. Because we know that physical activity is so beneficial, I have often been asked how one draws the line between a healthy amount of exercise and too much exercise. People with eating disorders may exercise excessively to try to control weight, and may develop health problems such as bone and heart problems. On the other hand, Olympic athletes certainly appear to have extreme work-outs. The important difference is that, instead of exercising for fitness or accomplishment, people with eating disorders who exercise excessively do so mainly for weight loss or to change their appearance, and will exercise even to the detriment of their health. They will do almost anything to maintain their exercise ritual and will become very distressed if they miss a work-out.

Traumatic events

Sometimes an eating disorder may be triggered by a traumatic life event, and a small percentage of patients with eating disorders have a history of being abused.

Dieting

Although most people who diet do not develop eating disorders, eating disorders often begin with a diet. People who develop anorexia nervosa begin dieting, and this escalates until they lose too much weight. Those with bulimia begin dieting and then develop a vicious cycle of binge eating and either purging, intermittent dieting, or excessive exercising.

Why Are Eating Disorders So Serious?

Eating disorders can affect one's physical health as well as one's mental health. They can also affect every other aspect of a person's life, including school, family and social life.

Medical complications

Eating disorders can affect almost every organ system in the body, and their effects can range from mild in some patients to extremely severe in others. With excessive weight loss or inadequate nutrition, as in anorexia nervosa, women can have irregular menstrual cycles or stop menstruating. Both males and females may develop bone thinning or bone loss, known as osteopenia or osteoporosis. This puts one at risk for developing bone fractures, especially in the hip and spine. Patients with anorexia nervosa lose muscle mass, including heart-muscle mass. This in turn can lead to a weakened heart. Additional complications include kidney problems, infertility, and gastrointestinal problems, among others. Patients with bulimia develop dental problems from erosion of tooth enamel from vomiting. They can also have electrolyte abnormalities from vomiting or using laxatives or diuretics, and this can lead to heart rhythm disturbances and even death. Irritation of the esophagus can result from acid damage due to vomiting, and some patients even develop tears of the esophagus. Patients with binge-eating disorder are also at risk and may have gastrointestinal problems as well as complications related to obesity.

Psychosocial complications

Medical problems are not the only concern when it comes to eating disorders. People with eating disorders are preoccupied with thoughts about food, weight and body shape. They often lack energy, have poor concentration, and almost always have low self-esteem. There is a higher incidence of depression, anxiety disorder, and obsessive-compulsive symptoms in people suffering from eating disorders. Many of these symptoms will improve, or even resolve, once the eating disorder is treated. People suffering from eating disorders find that all aspects of their lives—family, school or work and social—are affected.

Associated disorders

Certain psychiatric conditions may coexist in people with eating disorders. These include mood disorders, anxiety disorders, obsessive-compulsive disorder and personality disorders. Unfortunately, some people with eating disorders may abuse substances.

How Does One Recognize an Eating Disorder?

The following are some of the more specific clinical symptoms found in the various eating disorders.

Anorexia nervosa

Individuals with anorexia nervosa are underweight. Because of "lack of fuel" (inadequate calories), body functions slow down. This leads to a low body temperature, slow heart rate and low blood pressure. The person often feels cold all the time, and may notice the growth of fine hair over the face or body (lanugo hair). Girls who have begun menstruating will stop. Because of insufficient calories, people with anorexia nervosa have slowing down of the emptying of the stomach ("delayed gastric emptying") and may develop constipation or feel bloated after eating small amounts of food. Individuals with anorexia are preoccupied with dieting, weight and shape. They may feel weak and have difficulty concentrating.

Bulimia nervosa

People with bulimia nervosa have regular episodes of binge eating, and may diet between the binges. They are often of normal weight, or may even be slightly overweight. They are preoccupied with their body weight or shape and their weight may fluctuate frequently. They can develop calluses on their fingers, which are sometimes used to induce vomiting. Dental-enamel erosions may occur from acid damage. Patients may also complain of abdominal pain, sore throat or heartburn. Some develop swollen cheeks due to enlarged salivary glands (from vomiting repeatedly). Very often, the eating-disorder behavior causes shame and embarrassment and people may isolate themselves from their friends and even from family.

Binge-eating disorder

People with binge-eating disorder have regular episodes of binge eating, and may diet on and off. They are usually, but not always, overweight. Their symptoms may include abdominal pain, bloating, or constipation, or they may have symptoms related to obesity in general. Some may have a depressed mood or become socially isolated, and most people with binge-eating disorder have low self-esteem.

Do You Have an Eating Disorder?

You may, if you:

- Constantly worry about your weight or your body shape.
- Feel as if you have lost control over how much you eat.
- Diet regularly.
- Exercise excessively.
- Feel guilty about eating.
- Believe that you are fat even when others say you are thin.
- Have low self-esteem.
- Believe that how you look and how much you weigh is related to your value as a person.

If you think you may have an eating disorder, it is important to get help as soon as possible, as early appropriate treatment will improve the outcome. A good place to start is with your primary-care doctor, who will refer you to a treatment team if necessary (see below).

Treatment of Eating Disorders

Treatment for someone with an eating disorder includes some form of psychotherapy — individual, family, and/or group therapy — as well as medical management and nutritional counseling. In individuals who are significantly underweight, weight needs to be restored before meaningful therapy can be begun. Sometimes medication is used in addition to therapy to treat associated symptoms such as depression or anxiety. Medication may also decrease the urge to binge, and help prevent relapse in some patients. Treatment is usually best done by a team of healthcare providers familiar with treating people with eating disorders. The team may include a medical doctor, a psychiatrist, a registered dietitian, a psychologist, a licensed clinical social worker, and/or a nurse. Although eating disorders are serious illnesses, they are treatable.

15

Guide for Parents: Basic Strategies

If you are a parent of an overweight child, it is difficult to know how best to become involved. You have probably read about the serious health consequences of obesity and therefore know that you can't sit by idly and do nothing. On the other hand you may be apprehensive about approaching your child about weight issues, especially if he or she already has low self-esteem. A good place to start is by setting up a physical examination with your child's pediatrician, who can evaluate your child's weight, body-mass index and health in general. He or she will determine whether there is a problem, as well as the extent of the problem. The pediatrician can then make recommendations, or can refer you to a specialist or team of healthcare providers familiar with the treatment of obesity.

Having children assessed for weight problems is important because childhood is when we have the best chance of preventing obesity and its complications from progressing into adulthood. Also, being overweight can negatively affect the self-esteem of young people, so the earlier we address the problem, the better chance they have of developing good self-esteem. The most common cause of the recent increase in obesity is most likely lifestyle behaviors such as taking in too many calories and doing too little physical activity. However, it is important that the evaluation include looking for underlying medical and psychological problems that could contribute to eating and weight problems (see appendix B). Although rare, genetic and hormonal causes of obesity should be ruled out. The work-up should also include being assessed for eating disorders, as treatment may

differ. For example, someone with binge-eating disorder would usually benefit from therapy in addition to nutritional counseling.

Be aware that your child may have eating problems even if he
or she is not overweight. If you notice signs of disordered eating, or
are concerned that your child may have an eating disorder, check
with the primary-care doctor. The earlier an eating disorder is appropriately treated, the better the prognosis. For a discussion of the various eating disorders see the preceding chapter.

Could Your Child Have an Eating Disorder?

The following are some clues that might indicate an eating problem or eating disorder in your child.

- Regular episodes of overeating and/or feeling out of control over
  the eating behavior.
- Restrictive dieting behavior, or skipping meals.
- Marked fear of weight gain or of becoming fat.
- Feeling cold all the time.
- Extremely picky eating, or excluding certain food groups.
- Signs that your child may be vomiting or using pills in order to lose
  weight.
- Symptoms of depression, or isolation from family and friends.
- Refusal to eat meals with the family.
- Your child has poor body image and feels badly about the way he
  or she looks.
- Your child believes (s)he is fat even though (s)he is not.
- Your daughter has stopped menstruating or has irregular menstrual
  periods.
- Your child is overweight or underweight, or has had a rapid change
  in weight.
- His or her weight fluctuates markedly.

These symptoms can also be signs of other problems, so it is
important to have a thorough assessment.

Dealing with the Obesity Problem

Treatment of obesity usually includes medical monitoring, nutritional counseling, increasing physical activity (and decreasing inactivity), as well as therapy and medication if needed. Your primary-care physician can help decide which of these components of treatment are needed.

One mother's story

I spoke to a mother of a fifteen-year-old girl, who had been struggling to lose weight. "It's been so hard for Allie. She's tried various diets and nothing has helped. First she cut out sweets and cakes, but that lasted for only a short time. She then joined me on a low-carb diet, which we stayed on for six weeks. The problem was that when she came off the diet, she gained even more weight and became very frustrated. It seems as if she's lost all motivation now. Allie doesn't want to go to a gym because she is so embarrassed about her body, so she gets very little exercise."

I asked about her daughter's friends and social life. "Her friends really like her, but she doesn't see it that way. She won't believe that they can see past her weight. Recently Allie's been isolating herself more because there are so many activities she won't take part in. She won't go swimming, she won't go clothes-shopping, and lately she even avoids going out to eat with friends. Shopping for clothes is one of the most frustrating things for her. It's hard for her to find pretty clothes that fit. Most of the time Allie puts on a brave front and tells us that her weight doesn't bother her, but I know that inside she hurts a lot. I only wish I could help her more."

In this chapter I will discuss what you as parents can do to help and guide your children.

Mrs. Dawson's story—who's in charge here?

Mrs. Dawson took her thirteen-year-old son Mike to the pediatrician for a routine physical. Mike had been gaining weight steadily since he gave up sports the year before, and recently he had been spending most of his free time playing video games. His doctor told Mrs. Dawson that Mike was 40 pounds overweight, and that his cholesterol was very high. They were going to do further testing, which would include assessing for diabetes or pre-diabetes, but in the meantime it was essential that Mike make some lifestyle changes in order to lose weight. The complications of obesity were explained to Mike and his parents and they all seemed to understand. Mike was to spend less time playing video games and he and his family were to visit with a dietitian, develop healthier eating patterns, begin daily short walks, and return after two weeks.

The day before Mike's scheduled visit, Mrs. Dawson called to reschedule the visit for the following week. She said that it was difficult to get Mike to come in. When he did come in three weeks later, he had not made any of the suggested changes. He was also still spending most of his free time playing video games. Mr. and Mrs. Dawson said that they had no control over that.

I wanted to comment on this situation, because I see similar situations all the time. As parents, you do have some control over your child's health and healthy behaviors. Who better to teach them healthy habits? No, you can't and shouldn't force your child to eat something he doesn't want to eat, and you don't want to be the "food police." I don't believe in restricting your child from eating when he wants to eat. That can backfire, and lead to sneak eating or binge eating, and doesn't allow your child to understand his own hunger signals. However, you can make a house rule that limits the time spent watching television and playing video games. Parents can help a lot by modifying the home environment. For example, you can keep the television set in a less-desirable place in the house so that family members are less enticed to watch often. You can buy an exercise bike or other exercise equipment so that they will be more likely to exercise. You also have control over the quality of food kept in the home and money spent on fast foods and vending machines. Don't single your child out, but in a situation like this where health is on the line, develop a strategy that works for all of you. Consult with your child's primary-care doctor who can offer guidance. A good way to go is to make healthy changes that involve the whole family.

Pam's Story

Pam, mother of thirteen-year-old Katie, told me that her daughter has lost weight and is healthier today because she (Pam) realized that she was the one who needed to make some changes. For years Pam and her husband worried about Katie, the oldest of their three children. Katie spent hours a day watching television, rarely socializing with friends. She would eat when she was bored or lonely, and often would share chips or popcorn with her mother while watching their favorite shows together. Although her two brothers participated in sports, Katie was relatively inactive, and began gaining weight rapidly.

Her parents urged her to get help to improve her eating and to increase her physical activity, but Katie, vehemently denying that she had a problem, refused. Her parents felt helpless. Although her self-esteem was poor and she began isolating herself even more, the situation did not change until, at her routine check-up, Katie was found to have high cholesterol and insulin levels. Pam realized that her daughter was at risk for developing diabetes if she did not change her lifestyle habits. She made up her mind that although Katie had no motivation to change, she herself would make changes—changes that involved the whole family, and didn't single out Katie or focus on her weight. Everyone could benefit by eating more nutritiously and being more active. She made these family changes gradually. The first change involved television. She and her husband made a family rule limiting TV to no more than one- and-one-half hours a day. There was no mention of physical activity at that time, but Pam noticed that once family members were not watching as much TV, they started doing other things, such as reading, calling friends, or playing ball outside. The next change came two weeks later when she made a plan for the family to take walks together after dinner a few nights a week. At first everyone complained, but after the first week they started looking forward to the walks and the time spent together.

The most difficult change for Pam to make was giving up snacking with Katie while watching movies or TV shows. That habit was hard to break. It was their time together — their bonding time. Instead she decided to bond with Katie in other ways. Both mom and daughter were collectors. They set aside two hours on weekends and went to flea markets and garage sales together. They began collecting interesting items, and meeting interesting people. During the week, if Katie had free time, she would work on crafts and art projects she had picked up at the sales. This was so much more fun than watching TV — and what's more she was moving around, and didn't have time to think of snacking, because she wasn't bored. A few months later, everyone had made some changes. All family members were watching less TV, were walking five days a week, and were snacking less. Without focusing much on weight, Katie had lost several pounds, and was a happier and more active person.

You Help Determine Your Child's Eating Patterns and Weight

As a parent you do play a role in determining your child's eating patterns and lifestyle habits. You have some control over your child's exposure to the media and therefore to media messages of cultural ideals as well as numerous food advertisements on television. You also determine to some extent their meal portion sizes, whether they routinely have second helpings, and their ability to regulate their own food intake. For example, you can promote overeating by insisting that your child always "clean her plate." On the other hand, excessive restriction can also lead to overeating in the form of bingeing or sneak eating. It has been shown that when certain foods were restricted, children developed an increased preference for those foods, and, when able, ate more of them even when not hungry.

Get the whole family involved

If you want to change your child's eating or exercise behaviors, you are probably more likely to succeed if you do this as a family. This is particularly important if you have younger children or teenagers. A study comparing treatments of overweight children compared treating the child only, treating the child with the parents, or having no treatment at all. When children were treated alone, they were able to maintain weight, and when the whole family was treated, children lost weight. Without treatment, weight gain occurred.

Parents are very important role models. It may not always seem that way, but your children watch what you do and learn from your behaviors. If health and fitness is a priority to you, chances are that your child will adopt some of your healthy habits. Change your own eating behaviors and your children will change theirs. If your children see you watch television for hours every day, they may very well learn that habit from you. On the other hand, the best way to get your kids to watch less TV is to watch less yourself. A healthier lifestyle can benefit every family member. For a number of other reasons, it's also easier if everyone is involved. Your child won't feel singled out, and everyone will be able to eat the same foods, which means that you won't have to prepare different meals for different family members. Having family support and involvement can also be a good motivator. In short, establishing healthy eating and exercise habits for your family now will be one of the best things you can do to help them with lifelong weight and health management.

Don't scare your child

Even though you may be concerned about all the complications of obesity, be careful about how you approach your child. Scaring her probably won't help, and may even lead to dangerous dieting. Instead, promote gradual changes towards a healthier lifestyle for the whole family.

Promote Healthy Eating

Eating portions that are too large, eating high-calorie, high-fat foods, skipping breakfast, and drinking sodas and juices all contribute to excessive weight gain, especially when this is combined with more sedentary activity. The earlier you begin to teach your children how to eat in a healthy, balanced way, the better chance they will have of practicing long-term healthy eating habits.

What is healthy eating?

Eating in a healthy way means eating regular meals and snacks, usually three meals and one or two snacks a day. It also means eating a balance of foods from all the food groups— getting sufficient proteins and carbohydrates as well as fats. Dietary fats provide a number of important functions, including helping with the absorption of fat-soluble vitamins. The best kind of fats are unsaturated fats (found in foods such as olive oil, almonds, etc.), rather than saturated fats (found in foods like butter, cheese and whole milk.) A reasonable guideline is that no more than 30 percent of the day's calories should come from fat, and no more than 10 percent of the day's calories from saturated fat. (However, as a general rule, I don't recommend that fat intake be restricted in infants under the age of two years.) It's also important for children to get sufficient calcium in their diets. They can accomplish this by getting three servings of low-fat dairy products each day. If they don't get this, check whether they need a supplement. Recent focus on low-carb diets can be confusing. There is no need to try to eliminate carbohydrates. They are an important source of energy. Choose whole-grains such as whole wheat bread and brown rice over refined carbohydrates when you can. They are more nutritious and more filling.

Start them off right

Start teaching your children about healthy choices when they are very young. Make nutritious foods like fruits and vegetables familiar and a regular part of their diet. Teach them the importance of having a good breakfast. Eating breakfast will lessen the chance of excessive snacking later in the day. It also gives them energy and can help them concentrate. Teach them to eat regular meals and snacks and to appreciate foods that are good for them. If they don't become accustomed to eating fruits and vegetables regularly, get into the habit of eating at fast-food restaurants several times a week, and develop a taste for fried foods at an early age, chances are they will continue to eat this way when they are older. So, expose your children to lots of tasty healthy foods. Let them see you munching crunchy apples instead of chips for snacks, and when they are old enough to understand, let them know the benefits of these healthy habits.

Place emphasis on a healthy lifestyle rather than pressuring them to reach a certain size or weight. Focus on healthy eating rather than restrictive dieting. By dieting, your child may lose weight in the short term, but if she doesn't adopt new lasting habits, she will return to her previous lifestyle and probably regain that weight or more. This can lead to poor self-esteem, and can sometimes lead to eating disorders. Support your child in making gradual healthy lifestyle changes—one or two small ones at a time. When these become habit, move on to the next ones. All family members could be involved in making healthy changes. As a result of these healthy lifestyle habits, your child is likely to lose weight, but the first goal must be healthier eating and activity, and not weight loss.

Don't forbid certain foods or criticize your child for eating. Rather be supportive by limiting triggers of overeating such as leaving cookies on the kitchen table. There is no problem with snacking as long as one pays attention to the quality and the quantity of the snacks. Most children would benefit by having a planned healthy snack in the afternoon, for example. This breaks the long period of time between lunch and dinner and can prevent overeating later in the evening. The problem is that many children today snack on large amounts of high-fat, high-carbohydrate foods, which lead to excessive weight gain.

Teach your child to regulate herself. Serve nutritious foods at mealtimes, but once you have served them, let your child decide what and how much she wants to eat. This will help her develop her own hunger cues. If you do dish out servings, make sure the portion sizes are appropriate and not too large. Your child can always come back for more if she is still hungry. Studies show that people tend to eat in proportion to the amount that is served them, rather than how hungry they are. So, if you serve portions that are too large, you may be encouraging your child to eat more than she really wants. Make it easier for your child to eat healthily by making healthy snacks such as fruits and vegetables, low-fat dairy products, and whole grains available to them. Plan ahead for that after-school period when your child comes home hungry and will probably eat almost anything they find in the pantry. Put out a plate of cut-up apples, strawberries and yogurt, or whole-wheat crackers and peanut butter, instead of letting them snack on cookies and chips. Make smoothies by blending fresh fruits with low-fat yogurt or milk. Sodas and fruit juices contain a large number of calories, so discourage the drinking of sodas, and limit fruit juices. Cutting out one regular soda a day can lead to a large weight loss over a year. Ask all family members to be involved. Let all of them take turns coming up with suggestions for healthy meals and treats. Let your child help you with grocery shopping and with cooking. Most important of all, keep a positive attitude.

Eat meals together

It is sad that not enough families sit down to have at least dinners together. Meal-time can be such an important time to spend together and catch up on what's happening in your children's lives. It provides structure, and is also a critical time to shape your child's eating behaviors and to model healthy eating. It has been shown that children who eat meals with their families tend to eat healthier foods, and eat more fruits and vegetables. A common problem I see in both patients who are overweight as well as those with eating disorders is that their families don't eat together on a regular basis. Teenagers may rush in from school, grab something to eat on the run, and rush to an after-school activity. Some parents work late and so it is not feasible for children to wait until they return to eat dinner. Children may not always make the healthiest choices under those circumstances. I understand how difficult it is for two-career families—I am part of one. However, in most cases, it is worth the sacrifices you have to make to be able to share at least one meal a day with your children. If it can't be dinner, make it breakfast or lunch. If you can't get everyone together on a daily basis, plan to have meals together on weekends.

Make mealtimes pleasant. Let each family member share a good experience that occurred during the day, or you could even share a joke or two. Let them know that this family time is important to you. Always eat meals at the dining room or kitchen table, rather than making anywhere in the house an eating place. If you do return from work very late and have no other option, plan ahead so that your children can have a light healthy dinner at an earlier time, and then sit down with you for a few minutes and perhaps share some fruit and yogurt. I have included some ideas for easy dinners later in this book.

Promote Increased Physical Activity

Overweight children are often more sedentary than children who are not overweight. Exercising on a regular basis can help children lose weight and help them maintain their weight loss. Exercise has many other benefits, such as strengthening muscles including the heart muscle, and improving body image and self-esteem. Also, it has been shown that people can benefit from regular healthy physical activity even when they don't lose weight.

Become a more active family. Set up a regular activity, such as a family basketball match or taking a walk together in the evenings. On the weekend, go bowling, or consider going for a short hike and having a picnic, rather than driving to a restaurant for lunch. Schedule active family outings, for example to the zoo or to the beach. Encourage active play. Give your kids "activity gifts" such as a tennis lesson, a basketball, or tickets to go ice skating, rather than new video games. Set a good example by letting your children see you participate in regular physical activity. Let them also see you incorporate physical activity in your day-to-day life. Weed the garden, or take a walk to a friend's home instead of driving. Remember that it's always best to check with a physician to make sure that it is safe for each family member to participate in physical activity.

Aerobic activity

Children should participate in some form of aerobic activity on a regular basis. The new recommendations are that healthy people get about an hour of physical activity on most days. This does not mean they have to start out with an hour a day. Any amount of activity is better than no activity at all. So, if they have not been exercising regularly, starting out with five or ten minutes of light activity a day and gradually increasing time and intensity is fine. Also, this does not have to be structured exercise. Active play will also be beneficial. The important thing is that your children do something that they like to do, so that they are more likely to continue being active. A few examples of aerobic activities are walking, running, biking, skating, swimming, basketball, and dancing.

Strength training

Adding strength training (generally with weights) to an exercise routine can be beneficial. Strength training increases muscle strength. It also increases lean body mass, which increases metabolism and contributes to weight loss. It is very important for young people to be supervised when participating in strength training, so that they will learn good form and prevent injury. Children and adolescents should not participate in body-building, power lifting or competitive weight lifting until their bones reach maturity.

Set limits on media time

The more your child watches television, the more likely he or she will become overweight. There is a definite correlation between time spent watching television or participating in other sedentary behaviors, and obesity. Children who watch more than four hours of television a day tend to have a much higher body-mass index. Of course there is no need to stop your children from watching television, but the American Academy of Pediatrics recommends that you limit their media time to no more than one to two hours a day. Let your whole family make that commitment. It is also advisable to keep television out of their bedrooms (up to two-thirds of 8- to 18-year-olds have TV sets in their bedrooms!) and to discourage eating while watching TV. Watching less television will allow your children more time to be active, and will lessen their exposure to commercials promoting high-calorie, high-fat snack foods. Help your children find more creative ways to spend that time.

Set Realistic Goals

You can help your child set healthy goals. Setting specific goals such as weight loss is fine and can be motivating. However, help your child keep in mind that the main goal should be healthier eating and activity. Having him lose fifteen pounds on a drastic diet only to regain that weight or more is not a solution. Instead, you want to teach your child(ren) healthy principles that can last a lifetime. In this case, by making only a few simple changes, you can all be well on the way to achieving your goals. If your son or daughter is under the age of 14, you will be responsible for implementing and monitoring many of the lifestyle changes. It is not realistic to expect a 12-year-old to be committed enough to make significant lifestyle changes alone. Older adolescents can take on more of the responsibility, depending upon their degree of motivation. As you read earlier, some parents have told me that they have no control over how or what their child eats. That's not entirely accurate. You do have some control. You can start by keeping healthier foods in the house, by limiting sodas, and by eating out less often. You can also encourage family members to eat only in designated eating areas, and make a rule about not eating while watching television.

Help with Monitoring, but Don't Take Over

Monitoring is a powerful tool to help one become healthier and lose weight, help one maintain weight loss or just keep one on track. Recording weights at weekly or monthly intervals can help people keep track of their progress and can be a strong motivator. Detailing one's food intake and physical activity can be done by journaling daily. Encourage your child to monitor him- or herself and perhaps you can monitor yourself too. This is a way of showing support without making anyone feel singled out. If you have a young child who is not yet motivated to keep a food journal, ask if you can help do so.

Promote a Healthy Body Image and Good Self-esteem

Children really do learn from what they see around them. Before you can really address healthy body-image issues with your child, whether a son or a daughter, it is important that you take a look at your own beliefs and your own body image. Do you have a healthy body image? Do you believe that your self-worth is greater when you look a certain way or when you're thinner? If you do, that may affect the way your child feels. Your own eating behaviors and the way you feel (and what you say) about your own weight and body can have a significant effect on your child's eating habits, dieting behavior and body image. Set a good example for your children by accepting your own body, and by not judging people by their appearance. That does not mean that you can't all strive to be healthier by maintaining an active lifestyle and eating nutritious foods.

Be Supportive

It is better to be positive and supportive of your child rather than judgmental and critical. Unfortunately, overweight children are too often exposed to teasing, at school, on the streets, by strangers and even by friends. They often feel embarrassed and ashamed. Make your child feel loved, respected and secure. Let him know that you accept and love him no matter what he weighs. There is no place for teasing at home. Home should be a place where your child always feels safe. A child who feels criticized for being overweight may rebel by eating more.

Spend time with your children and really listen to them, and praise them for good values, effort and for accomplishments unrelated to appearance.

Weight-Loss Camps

An option that is available to children and teenagers struggling with their weight is a summer camp that focuses on nutrition, fitness and weight loss. In an ideal camp situation, children should be taught healthy eating and activity habits, meet friends, gain self-confidence, and have fun. They should also feel supported. The downside is that although campers do adopt healthier habits and lose weight in the structured camp environment, if they return to their old habits, they will quickly regain that weight when they return home. That can lead to frustration and poor self-esteem.

On the positive side, however, I do think there is a place for camps that focus on lifestyle behaviors, fitness and nutrition. Children have an opportunity to learn about health and life skills and to participate in a variety of physical activities. They are also surrounded by other young people with similar concerns. The best camps are those that emphasize long-term (healthy) behavioral change, involve families to some extent, and provide access to follow-up programs.

There's No Need for Perfection

Remember that there's no need for you or for your child to be perfect. No one is. If you don't always reach the goal you set out to achieve, that's okay, as long as you are making some strides towards it. Even small positive changes can make a big difference.

16

Guide for Parents: Focus on Food

How One Mother Made a Difference

Janice, a mother of three young school-children, was concerned about the quality of her kids' school lunch program. She thought that the lunches their private school offered were much too high in fat and sugar and lacked fruits and vegetables. In that respect she was much like the other parents at the school. The difference was that she not only complained, she also took bold steps to do something about the problem.

Janice began by spending time in the cafeteria at lunch. She watched the kids wait in long slow lines for French fries, burgers, fried chicken and mashed potatoes. By the time they received their food, they had only a few minutes to swallow it and then had to rush back to class. Sometimes they had enough time to grab a few cookies and a juice or soda on their way. The children seemed rushed and irritable. What she saw certainly could not be described as a relaxing lunch break.

Janice applied to be in charge of the lunch program for the following year, and the position was granted to her. She began by hiring a new chef, and staggering lunch times, so that the students would not have to wait in line so long. She told the staff that she wanted to change the menu entirely. Instead of fried chicken, burgers and fries, she wanted options such as grilled chicken, baked potatoes, vegetables, and turkey or vegetable wraps. Rather than offering chips and cookies for dessert, she would make yogurts and cut-up pears, strawberries, kiwis and mangoes available. The administration and many parents were skeptical. "Children wouldn't be happy with this drastic change," they said. "They'd be upset if they couldn't eat fries and hamburgers at lunch. They'd miss cookies for dessert. No one would choose fruit."

Janice stood her ground. The new chef turned out to be excellent, and not only prepared healthy foods, but presented them beautifully. The kids, although concerned about the change at first, were happily surprised by how good the food tasted. They were also relieved to have more time to eat. They seemed less hurried. Soon they were looking forward to seeing what was on the lunch menu, and were enjoying sampling the colorful fresh fruits.

Who says that children don't know what's best for them?

How You Can Make a Difference

Here are some practical "dos and don'ts" for parents who want their families to be healthy.

What to do

Stock the fridge and pantry with healthy foods that taste good. Plan menus in advance and ask your child to help with planning and preparing meals.

Offer a variety of healthy choices at meals, but let your child decide how much he or she wants to eat.

When cooking, grill, bake or poach, rather than fry or sauté. Try to cut down on creamy sauces and gravies. Remove the skin and fat from chicken and meat before cooking. Offer everyone water instead of sodas and high-calorie juices.

Eat meals together with your children when possible. Consider starting meals with a healthy salad or broth-based soup to fill them up and make them less likely to overeat later. Because it takes time to feel satisfied, eating more slowly may prevent overeating.

Encourage family members to eat mindfully. In other words, when you eat, concentrate on eating and enjoying your food. Don't watch television or do other things while you eat.

What not to do

Although it's important to guide your children, don't be too controlling over what and how much they eat. In other words, don't force your children to eat when they are not hungry and don't withhold food when they are hungry. They need to learn to develop their own hunger and satiety cues and to regulate their eating. Restricting intake when they want to eat may also lead them to feel guilty about eating.

Note: In certain situations such as anorexia nervosa, parents frequently do need to help with refeeding their sick child who is not paying attention to his or her own hunger cues.

Don't offer sweets, or any other food, as a reward. Food should not be a substitute for attention or love. A far better reward would be time spent together. Children have told us so!

Don't promote dieting behavior. Many young people who diet continue to develop yo-yo dieting, or binge eating, and may even gain more weight. One large study showed that teenagers who dieted often were more likely to become overweight.

Don't talk about good or bad foods. That again can lead to feelings of guilt once a food in the "bad" category has been eaten. Most foods, within reason, can fit in to a healthy eating plan.

Don't tolerate teasing about weight or appearance. Be clear that this includes teasing each other as well as talking about others, even when they are not present. Hearing disparaging remarks made about overweight people in general can leave an overweight child feeling badly about him- or herself.

Family Behavior Checklist

Answer "yes" or "no" to the questions on the list below and see how your family fares now. Revisit it in a month's time and note whether there are any improvements.

1. Family members eat at least three meals a day.
2. Family members eat meals together at least once a day on average.
3. Television time is limited to no more than one to two hours a day.
4. Eating takes place in designated eating areas such as the dining room or the kitchen, and not the bedroom or in front of the TV.
5. Children are encouraged to eat and exercise for health rather than only to reach a certain size or weight.

6. Family members eat at least five servings of fruits and vegetables daily.
7. Family eats out or orders take-out no more than three times a week.
8. Family members do some form of physical activity for at least a half-hour on most days.
9. Family members share some form of physical activity or an active hobby at least once a week (this may include a walk together).
10. Food is not used as a reward.
11. Teasing about size or weight is not tolerated.

Give yourself one point for every question checked off as "yes."

If you scored:

9–11: Your family is doing really well with respect to lifestyle behaviors. Keep it up!

6–8: There is room for improvement. Review the suggestions in the book and see if you can make any positive changes within the next month.

0–5: Changes are needed. Your family is not unusual, as many families are busy and find it difficult to sit down to meals together, eat on the run, and feel as if they have no time for physical activity. Work together with your family to make gradual healthy changes that will benefit everyone.

If we do nothing about the "overweight crisis," the problem is only going to get worse. More children will become overweight and in turn will grow up to become adults who are overweight. We should not panic, but we should take some action now.

When Things Aren't Going Well:

As a parent, you may feel as if you have done all that can be done, and yet you still see no positive changes. What could be going on?

Problems with monitoring

Monitoring is a powerful tool in the treatment of weight problems, as it can help identify poor eating habits and insufficient physical activity. However, if your child is not monitoring accurately, this will not be very helpful. I have seen several patients bring in food diaries reflecting calorie intakes of only 1000 or 1200 calories a day, but instead of losing weight, they were gaining weight. This was all a result of inaccurate recording. You can help your child by encouraging her to record her intake at least daily, or even after each meal. Try to present this in a supportive way, rather than being critical. Another problem may be poor recording of portions. In order for a dietitian to make an assessment of calorie intake, a reasonable idea of portion sizes will be necessary. So, although you do not need to count calories, it will be important to indicate the approximate portions of foods and beverages. Eating a soup bowl of ice cream is very different from eating a "dish" of ice cream.

Lack of motivation

Although you can not afford to do nothing if your child is overweight, success becomes much more likely if he or she is motivated to change. Constantly pushing someone who is unwilling to change can lead to repeated failures and a damaged self-esteem. Sometimes a child who was motivated at first can become unmotivated during the treatment process. One reason may be that progress may be too slow. He may have expected faster results with respect to weight loss or fitness, or even social changes. He may also find it difficult not to eat as his friends do, and may struggle with self-control. You and the physician can help overcome these problems by setting smaller, attainable goals, and by positive reinforcement of healthy lifestyle behaviors.

Ineffective routine

I know of someone who worked out at a health club almost every day. The problem was that she developed the routine of meeting her friend at the club cafeteria after every workout session. Together they chatted over dessert or a milkshake. Your child could be exercising on a regular basis, but she could be undoing much of her hard work if she rewards her daily effort with an extra dessert.

Saboteurs

Although this may seem hard to believe, sometimes not everyone in the family wants to change. They may also not believe that it is in their best interests to have the patient make changes or lose weight. I spoke to a family in which the mother admitted that it was most difficult for her, because she and her daughter bonded best over eating. Her intentions were not bad. A family member may not understand the importance of making changes, and may unintentionally sabotage progress by keeping unhealthy tempting foods in the house. *Often the cook feels rewarded when the family members eat a lot.* Your child may also have a friend who feels threatened by your child's attempt at weight loss. This may be more likely to happen if the friend has eating issues herself. In this case, although she may eat very little herself, she may encourage your child to eat more or continually offer temptation. Not all family members and friends may be as supportive as they should be, and some may undermine treatment by teasing. All of these things can stand in the way of a good outcome.

Negative reinforcement

I believe that positive reinforcement works best when trying to achieve good long-term results. Negative reinforcement, such as scolding your child for eating candy, may seem to work in the short term, but it may increase behaviors such as sneaking and hiding food, and binge eating. If your child does not seem to be making healthy lifestyle changes, re-examine whether you are using positive reinforcement appropriately.

Practical Tips for Healthy Food Shopping

Sample shopping list (make copies for yourself and take one along when you go shopping):

- Fresh fruits.
- Fresh vegetables—include cut-up carrots and cucumbers for easy school lunches.
- Low-fat or non-fat dairy products including milk, yogurt, cottage cheese and other cheeses.

- Eggs or Egg-beaters.
- High-fiber, unsugared cereals such as shredded wheat, Chex and Kashi cereals.
- Whole-grain products such as whole-wheat bread, whole-wheat pasta, brown rice and whole-wheat flour.
- Dried peas, beans and lentils for soups or stews.
- Turkey, skinless chicken, lean cuts of meat, fish.
- Healthy snacks such as dried fruits, almonds, raisins, granola, peanut butter.
- Low-fat dips and salsa.
- Applesauce or apple butter to substitute for butter or margarine when baking.
- Low-fat or fat-free frozen yogurt.
- Popcorn kernels for air-popping, or microwave popcorn (no more than 2 grams of fat per serving).
- Spices to add flavor and interest to meals.
- Olive oil and cooking sprays.
- Bottles of water or sugar-free flavored waters for school lunches.

Dinner Ideas for the Family:

Dinner 1

Salad with chopped lettuce, cucumber, red and yellow peppers, green onions and a vinaigrette dressing.
Grilled chicken or barbequed chicken.
A sweet potato and corn.
A half-cup of low-fat frozen yogurt.

Dinner 2

Tomato, green pepper and cucumber salad, with a little lemon, salt and pepper to taste.
Grilled or baked salmon with rosemary, lemon and pepper (no oil necessary).
Red potatoes and green beans.
Fruit salad.

Dinner 3

Broth-based soup.
Salad with tomato, fresh mozzarella cheese and basil.
Vegetarian chili served over brown rice.
Sorbet or sherbet.

Dinner 4

Green salad with olive oil and vinegar.
Oven-baked chicken with onions and green peppers in a tomato-based sauce (brown chicken in whole-wheat flour or bread crumbs before baking).
Brown rice.
One or two home-made oatmeal-raisin cookies (use whole-wheat flour, and substitute applesauce for some of the butter or margarine).

Dinner 5

Grilled chicken salad — Large mixed-green salad, with cut-up vegetables and pieces of grilled chicken, balsamic vinaigrette dressing (almonds optional).
Banana split with banana (slit length-wise), fat-free frozen yogurt, cut-up strawberries and a small amount of strawberry sauce (or strawberry purée).

Dinner 6

Spinach salad with red onions and mandarins or orange segments.
Whole-wheat soft taco wraps filled with grilled chicken, brown rice, salsa, and a small amount of avocado.
Assorted cut-up fresh fruits.

Guide for Eating Out

Eating outside of the home does not necessarily have to ruin a healthy eating plan, but it does make it more difficult. Studies show that children who ate out or ordered fast foods several times a week had a higher incidence of obesity. If you do go out to eat, choose restaurants that offer healthy choices and set an example for your child by ordering grilled or baked foods instead of fried foods, and limiting sodas and high-fat appetizers. Share portions or take half home if they are too large.

Guide for School Lunches

Sending your child to school with a "brown-bag" lunch may be a better bet than letting him eat in the school cafeteria and from the vending machine. You will be able to ensure that lunch is a balanced meal, you will save money, and your child will save time by not having to stand in cafeteria lines. Try to make lunches creative and tasty. Include some protein (such as turkey breast, grilled chicken, hummus (chick-peas), or hard-boiled egg), a fruit and a vegetable, and perhaps a low-fat dairy product such as yogurt or cottage cheese. If their lunches are not boring, they will be less likely to supplement them with snacks from the vending machine or the cafeteria.

Remember that you can't have complete control over what your children eat and how much exercise they do, nor should you want to. As they get older they won't be spending as much time at home. However, by teaching them good nutrition habits and the importance of a healthy lifestyle now, and by making them aware of the dangers of restrictive dieting, you will be laying a good foundation for the future. Hopefully they will choose to adopt those healthy habits forever.

17

Prevention

Prevention is far easier and far better than treatment when it comes to obesity (and eating disorders). Treatment is difficult, expensive, and not always successful. Also, if treatment is not started early enough, complications may have already occurred. It is worth, therefore, considering prevention strategies in everyone from an early age, and to improve nutrition and increase physical activity with the goal of staying healthy and preventing obesity. Once you do have weight problems they should be addressed as early as possible.

What You Can Do

1. Whether or not you are overweight, learn to eat in a healthy way. This means eating regular meals and not skipping meals, eating when you are hungry and stopping when you are full, and eating a variety of foods so that you have a well-balanced diet.
2. Move your body. Make physical activity a regular part of your life.
3. Forget the "diet" mentality. Diets that are too restrictive can be harmful. At best you will be hungry, and become frustrated when you regain the weight; at worst, you will develop health problems, including nutritional deficiencies or even eating disorders. It has been shown that teenage girls who diet frequently are more likely to become overweight.
4. Be proactive in your school by demanding healthier nutrition options and mandatory physical education.
5. Don't tolerate prejudice, teasing, or stereotyping on the basis of size or weight.
6. Lighten up mentally! You've probably realized that it's easier to

take care of your health when you're happier and not stressed. You will be more likely to eat in a healthy way, and physical activity will be more enjoyable. You can lighten up mentally by developing a positive attitude. Replace negative thoughts with positive ones. Spend time with people with whom you feel comfortable. And don't take yourself too seriously. Leave some time for fun!

What Parents Can Do

1. Be a good role model by modeling good behaviors with respect to eating, television-viewing and physical activity. If you watch hours of TV each day, how can you expect your child not to? If you practice unhealthy eating habits, your children are likely to do so too. I know of a teenager who was struggling to lose weight while his father, who was also overweight, ate hamburgers and fries several nights a week. It was no surprise that his son could not be motivated. Children do learn from what they observe.
2. Make it a priority to have meals together when possible. Children who eat meals with their families are more likely to eat healthier meals.
3. Starting when they're young, teach your children about healthy nutrition and healthy food choices. Encourage all family members to eat regular meals and snacks and get adequate amounts of calcium-rich food and at least five servings of fruits and vegetables a day. You can help them do this by ensuring that there are always healthy foods in the house and by gently guiding their choices.
4. Promote physical activity for the whole family. Plan fun, active outings. Instead of making short trips by car, consider making them by foot. Is it safe for your children to walk to school? Perhaps you could even walk with them.
5. Schedule check-ups with your child's pediatrician at least annually, and have his or her body mass index assessed. I don't believe that children should be weighed and measured in school. I think this can lead to further stigmatization of overweight children.
6. Let your child know that one's value as a person is not related to one's appearance.

7. Expectant mothers—Studies indicate that children who were breast-fed may be less likely to become obese, so consider this when deciding whether to breast- or bottle-feed.

What Society Can Do

1. Don't tolerate teasing or prejudice based on size or weight.
2. Advocate for responsible media and the marketing and promotion of healthy food choices and increased physical activity. Encourage a ban on "junk-food" advertising on children's television programs.
3. Demand television shows that portray young men and women more realistically. View the media critically when it comes to images of unrealistic, super-thin models and actresses and super-muscular actors.
4. Promote increased funding for research in the field of childhood obesity.
5. Encourage organizations and insurance companies to provide insurance coverage for the prevention and treatment of obesity and obesity-related illnesses and complications.
6. Lobby for healthier school nutrition programs. Advocate for healthy school lunches.
7. Lobby for mandatory daily physical education for children in kindergarten through 12th grade.
8. Lobby against fast-food restaurants (with high-calorie, high-fat options) in hospitals and schools.

What Teachers, Counselors and Coaches Can Do

1. Advocate for a healthier lifestyle for students, through healthier nutrition and more physical activity. Be aware of the dangers of restrictive dieting in young people.
2. Focus on healthy habits rather than on weight. Be cautious about comments related to weight.

In summary, there is no one thing that anyone can do to prevent children and teenagers from becoming overweight, but together we can make a big difference.

18

Questions, Answers and a Quiz

1. Q: There are so many diets and diet books out there. It gets really confusing. Just when I think I know what's healthy, I hear different advice. How can one sort this all out and know what to believe?
A: You're absolutely right. It does get confusing. Although there is a lot of good information available, unfortunately you will also find advice that is not accurate. The good news is that your pediatrician and a registered dietitian should be able to answer your nutrition questions and advise you on whether a plan is or is not safe to follow.

2. Q. What is healthier — a high-protein, low-carbohydrate diet or a low-fat diet?
A: The answer lies somewhere in the middle. You will probably lose weight on any diet that restricts calories, but that may not be the healthiest plan to follow. The key is to find a healthy way of eating that can last for your lifetime. You will not find this in any fad diet. To be healthy, you need adequate amounts of protein, fats and carbohydrates, and taking in too little or too much of any of these can lead to health problems.

3. Q: I have been exercising regularly on three days a week for the past two months, and have only lost one pound. I am discouraged and wonder why I am not losing more weight.
A: Although exercise is a very important part of a weight-loss program, you are more likely to lose weight if you also change your eating habits. Make a point of recording everything you eat and

drink for at least a week. You may not be fully aware of what you are eating unless you write it down. Take note of hidden sources of calories such as sodas and other drinks, salad dressings and sauces, and snacks. You can also accelerate your weight loss and fitness level by gradually increasing the frequency and the intensity of your physical activity. Consider exercising on an additional day or two a week, and if you find the activity too easy, "pump up" the intensity a little.

4. Q: I am very concerned about gaining weight and becoming fat. Is it reasonable to weigh myself daily?
   A: Because weight normally fluctuates from day to day, it is best to weigh yourself less frequently. Weighing yourself weekly in the morning before breakfast will be a good way to monitor your weight.

5. Q: I am trying to lose about ten pounds. Do I need to give up all sweets and desserts?
   A: No, that is not necessary. It is best not to deprive yourself of all the foods you enjoy. If you do, you will probably develop cravings for those foods, and this may even precipitate bingeing. Eat those treats occasionally and in small amounts. Remember, it's not only what you eat that counts, but also how much of it and how often.

6. Q: Is it safe to exercise when I am sick?
   A: It is probably fine to exercise with a mild cold, but if you have fever, pain, dizziness or a more serious infection, it is best to hold off on exercise, and check with a doctor.

7. Q: I am about thirty pounds overweight. I began menstruating about a year and a half ago. My menstrual periods have never been regular. Sometimes they are very heavy and sometimes I skip a month altogether. Do I need to worry?
   A: It's quite common to have irregular menstrual periods initially, although they usually do begin regulating within a year or so. Some people who are overweight and have irregular periods have a condition known as polycystic ovary syndrome (see chapter 2). It's worthwhile checking with your doctor.

8. Q: I've always thought I should avoid peanut butter because it is fattening, and now I read that it is healthy. What's the deal with peanut butter?

   A: Peanut butter or peanuts can be included in your diet even if you are trying to lose weight. Peanut butter contains protein and fiber (about 2 grams per 2 tablespoons), and although it does contain fat, it is mostly unsaturated fat, the type that is healthier for you. The key is to eat peanuts or peanut butter in moderation because they do provide substantial calories. A reasonable amount for a snack would be 2 tablespoons of peanut butter or a small handful of peanuts.

9. Q: If I eat a very-low-fat diet, am I guaranteed to lose weight?

   A: Not necessarily. In order to lose weight, you'll have to cut down on your total calorie intake in addition to fat intake, or increase your physical activity. Going on a low-fat diet does have health benefits, though, and can protect against heart disease. Fats provide more calories per gram than do carbohydrates or proteins, (9 calories per gram, versus 4 calories per gram) so you will be able to fill up on more (other) foods by eating less fat.

10. Q: I have lost quite a lot of weight over the last few months by cutting down on sweets and fats. Recently though I seem to be stuck at my present weight and I still have about 10 pounds to lose. Is there anything I can do to speed up my weight loss?

    A: You didn't mention exercise. If you are not exercising on a regular basis, start adding exercise into your daily routine. This will boost your metabolism and help you lose that extra weight. If you are already physically active, adding a few more minutes to your routine, or working out at a higher intensity, may be all that you need. By the way there is no need to exercise for more than an hour a day, unless you are training for a specific event, a marathon or the Olympics.

11. Q: I need a breakfast alternative to cereal. All my friends eat cereal for breakfast, but I don't like cereal and I don't like milk.

    A: Some other options for breakfast include the following: omelet made with three egg whites or one whole egg and two egg whites, mixed with vegetables; whole-wheat bagel or English muffin, with light or fat-free cream cheese and a fruit; smoothie made with fat-free yogurt or frozen yogurt, crushed ice, bananas and strawberries; pancakes topped with fresh fruit; slice of whole-wheat toast and a hard-boiled egg or an egg-white omelet; fruit salad or melon and a low-fat or fat-free yogurt.

12. Q: Is it okay to eat five times a day instead of having only three meals a day?
    A: Depending on your schedule and on your activity level, it may make a lot of sense to have five smaller meals a day instead of three larger ones. This will spread out your meals and prevent you from getting too hungry and overeating. Remember, though, that it is still the total number of calories that you eat each day that counts. So, if you are having five meals instead of three, make them smaller meals.

13. Q: I am eighteen years old and am at a healthy weight. Both my parents are overweight. Does this mean that I will become overweight?
    A: If both your parents are overweight, you have a higher risk of becoming overweight. However, the fact that you are already eighteen and still of normal weight makes it less likely. Also, even people who are genetically predisposed to obesity can offset their risk by eating healthily and exercising regularly. So, even though you are not overweight, keep yourself healthy by following a healthy nutrition plan and getting some form of exercise on most days.

14. Q: I eat very well during the day, but I develop cravings for sweets or cookies in the evenings after dinner. I usually give in to the cravings, and once I start, I usually eat too much. Any suggestions?
    A: Make sure that you are getting enough calories and a balanced diet during the day. Are you having a good breakfast? Eating too little in the daytime, or skipping meals, can set you up for hunger and cravings later on. If you are getting enough to eat during the day, and you crave something sweet after dinner, allow

yourself something small. Decide in advance what you will allow yourself to eat and make sure that you have those foods in the house. Then get rid of all the sweets and chocolates that tempt you to eat too much. If you want something sweet, consider dried fruit, low-fat frozen yogurt or a smoothie, a cup of sugar-free jello topped with a spoonful of whipped topping, frozen pieces of fruit such as grapes, or a low-fat hot chocolate drink made with skim milk. If you want something salty or crunchy, consider air-popped popcorn or pretzels. Sometimes just warm herb tea will do the trick. If you still crave those cookies, and have to keep them in the house, buy them in small packages, so that you have only one or two. Having a big open bag of cookies will be too tempting. Once you've had your evening snack, brush your teeth, read or do another activity, or go to bed. Have a good breakfast the next morning.

15. Q: Is it okay to use non-caloric sugar substitutes?
    A: Many foods we eat contain sugar substitutes. Remember that although the substitute may not contain many calories, the foods containing them may still be high in calories. So, check the label to make sure that it's worth substituting the food for the regular version. Refer to the warning labels on these products when applicable. For example, some products contain phenylalanine, which should be avoided by people who have a genetic condition known as phenylketonuria. Lastly, it's important to develop a preference for healthy natural foods, so if you are going to use sugar substitutes, keep them to a minimum.

16. Q: Will I lose weight faster if I become a vegetarian?
    A: Not necessarily. Many of the foods included in a vegetarian diet are high in calories and fat. Of course, if you eat large amounts of cookies and sweets, you will probably gain weight. Also, even though cheese, soy, nuts and peanut butter can be included in a healthy diet, they should be eaten in moderation.

17. Q: Will I become overweight if I eat at fast-food restaurants?
    A: Not necessarily, if you eat fast foods only occasionally and if

you choose healthier options like the burger without the mayonnaise and fries, and the salad bar. However, studies show that people who eat fast foods regularly tend to eat more calories, more sugar and more fat, and less fruits and vegetables than those who don't eat fast foods regularly. Fast foods are also frequently served in large portions. All of these factors may put one at increased risk for becoming overweight.

18. Q: I have been started on a medication to help me lose weight. To what extent do I still need to pay attention to what I eat and how much I exercise?
A: Medications to treat obesity should only be used together with physical activity and healthy eating to lose weight and maintain that weight loss long term. They should not take the place of healthy lifestyle changes.

19. Q: I eat healthily. I run on the treadmill for a half-hour on six days a week, and also do weight training on three days. I have lost weight, but that seems to have reached a plateau now. How can I change my exercise routine to get to the next level of fitness and possibly lose more weight?
A: First of all, you should think about alternating your running with another aerobic activity. Running is an excellent sport, but if you run on consecutive days, you run the risk of developing an overuse injury, such as shin splints. Why don't you consider running on three days of the week and alternating this with an activity such as biking or rowing? This way you will be using different muscles, and will be able to push yourself a little harder. It will also prevent you from getting bored with your routine.

20. Q: I have a family history of osteoporosis. Is there anything I can do to keep my bones strong and prevent osteoporosis?
A: Maintaining a healthy weight and getting enough calcium in your diet are two of the most important factors in preventing osteoporosis. You can get calcium by eating a variety of low-fat dairy products including milk, yogurt and cheeses. It's also important to participate in regular weight-bearing activities such

as running, basketball or dancing (among other choices). Avoid smoking and limit your intake of carbonated sodas.

21. Q: I follow a vegan diet and don't drink cow's milk, or eat cheese or yogurt. Where else can I get calcium, other than in calcium supplements?
A: You can get calcium by drinking calcium-fortified orange juice or rice or soy milk, or by eating vegetables like broccoli and kale.

22. Q: I am trying to support my fifteen-year-old daughter in her weight loss efforts, but I feel as if I have no control over how much she eats.
A: You shouldn't have to control how much your child eats. As a parent you should be responsible for providing your child with healthy meals and snacks, and should limit the availability of high-calorie, less-nutritious foods in the home. However, your child should decide how much food she wants to eat.

23. Q: What drinks can I pack for school lunch? I am trying to cut down on sodas.
A: Instead of soda, healthier options would be fat-free or low-fat milk, or water. Juices made from real fruits are an alternative, but it's better to eat the whole fruit (and to drink water) than to drink juice. Fruits provide fiber and will fill you up more.

24. Q: I was told not to lift weights if I want to lose weight, so that I would avoid "bulking up." Is that correct?
A: A moderate strength-training or weight-lifting program can actually help you maintain or even lose weight, as muscle burns more calories than fat. If you do lift weights or do any form of strength training, it's important that you be well supervised and use proper technique to avoid injury. It's also best to combine strength training with some form of aerobic activity on several days a week (e.g. biking, walking, dancing, etc.).

25. Q: I've always tried to avoid dairy products such as cheese, yogurt, ice cream and milk, because I thought they were fattening. Will staying off milk products help me lose weight?

A: There is no need to give up dairy products. Apart from being an excellent source of calcium, low-fat or non-fat dairy products such as yogurt, cheese or skim milk may actually help prevent weight gain. Teenagers should aim to get three servings of milk products daily. If you can't have dairy products, you can get calcium from other sources such as kale, canned salmon, fruit juice (fortified with calcium) or a calcium supplement.

26. Q: I am fifteen years old and fifty pounds overweight. I have been quite inactive for the past year, and want to start doing more physical activity. How should I begin? I don't belong to a gym, and I can't afford to buy any expensive equipment.
    A: Start by having a check-up with your primary care doctor. Make sure that it is safe for you to begin an exercise program. Walking is an excellent form of physical activity. You will be able to pace yourself so that you can slow down or stop if you feel tired. It can be done on your own, or you can choose to walk with a friend. You don't need any special equipment other than good walking shoes, and you don't need a gym. It might be fun and motivating to strap on a pedometer and measure how many steps you take each day.

True/False Quiz

Record your answers to these 10 true/false questions and then compare them to the correct answers given.

1. I should try to get at least five servings of fruits and vegetables a day.
2. A healthy person should get at least one-half to one hour's worth of physical activity on most days.
3. Skipping breakfast will help me save calories and achieve long-term weight loss.
4. By eating only one extra donut every day, I could gain an extra 25 pounds a year.
5. If both my parents are overweight, I should be resigned to the fact that I will be overweight.

6. Getting enough calcium in the form of low-fat dairy products can help protect against osteoporosis, and may aid in weight loss.
7. Watching more than two hours of television a day will increase my chances of becoming overweight.

Answers to quiz: 1. T 2. T 3. F 4. T 5. F 6. T 7. T

19

Conclusion

Obesity is a serious problem facing young people in the United States today, with 15 percent of children and teenagers now being classified as overweight or obese. None of us can afford to look the other way, because obesity comes with a high price to pay — in the form of medical and psychological complications, as well as social implications and a great financial burden. You are not alone if you have been confused about all the conflicting advice about how to manage your weight, or if you have secretly wished that the latest popular diet were the magic answer. If you are overweight, however, you don't have to feel overwhelmed. You also don't need to starve yourself or go on a fad diet to lose weight. This will only lead to frustration, "yo-yo dieting," and possibly even an eating disorder.

Many weight-loss books on the market promise a quick fix, a "magic" solution — or a special formula that will make the weight drop off. Well, I have to tell you something different. There is no quick fix, and there probably never will be a magic formula. Even when a more effective medication is approved (and it may be) you will still need to make those basic changes with respect to eating better and doing more physical activity in order to lose weight safely and have lasting health benefits.

Don't be disheartened, because this is a positive thing. By making gradual, healthy, permanent changes in your eating and exercise habits, you will feel better, be stronger and become healthier, and you will avoid the frustration that comes with trying one diet after another. Also, your weight loss will be maintained over the long term. As a teenager, you are in a good position to make these changes now, so that you can instill healthy habits early on, and try to avoid the serious complications seen too often in adults with obesity. It may be difficult in the beginning, but once you have taken the first step, the next step will become easier.

Our environment and our lifestyles have changed, in terms of nutrition, physical activity, usage of energy-saving devices, and lack of free time, and it's up to our whole society to work together to create a healthier environment. I believe that there is no need to blame any group for the obesity crisis, because we were all blind-sided by it, and could never have foreseen the extent of the problem. On the other hand, we do need to work together to make changes: — at home, in the school system, in restaurants, and in our government policies. We can't change everything at once, so why don't you start by doing what you can do. Hopefully this book can help you learn some ways to make healthy changes that you can live with. Changing your lifestyle habits should not be a short-term goal to change your appearance, but rather a lifelong way of living in order to become fitter and healthier. That will yield far more rewards than will a "magic pill."

Appendix A:
The Essentials of a
Healthier Lifestyle

Eat Better

- Eat balanced meals, and aim for a wide variety of nutritious, tasty foods.
- Eat three meals (including breakfast) and one or two small snacks each day.
- Stay away from restrictive dieting.
- Make sure you get enough fiber in your diet by eating at least five servings of fruits and vegetables every day, as well as foods such as whole grains, beans and peas.
- Get an adequate amount of calcium. You can achieve this by eating approximately three servings of low-fat or non-fat dairy products daily.
- Limit your intake of total and saturated fat.
- Choose complex carbohydrates over simple (refined) carbohydrates.
- Drink water or low-fat or non-fat milk instead of soft drinks or juices.
- Try not to think of foods as "good" or "bad" foods. Most foods are fine in moderation.

Be More Active

- Check with your physician before starting an exercise program.
- Aim to get about one hour of physical activity on most days. If you

have not been exercising regularly, it is fine to start with a few minutes and gradually work up to more.
- Choose activities you enjoy, and vary them.
- Set fitness goals and challenge yourself regularly.
- Add activity into your daily routine, such as taking the steps instead of the elevator, helping around the house, or walking to school instead of driving.

Be Less Inactive

- Limit media (including television) time to no more than one to two hours a day. When you do watch television, get up and move around during commercial breaks.
- Monitor how much time you spend at the computer, watching videos or movies, and playing video games.
- Instead of taking short trips in the car, consider making them by foot.

Monitor Yourself

- Weigh yourself weekly, preferably in the morning before eating.
- Record everything you eat and drink in a daily food diary to help you keep aware of your intake and your progress.
- Record the number of minutes you spend doing physical activity each day.
- Set goals for yourself and write them down. Re-evaluate them from time to time.
- Reward yourself in small ways when you reach your goals.

Reduce Your Stress

Learn ways to manage stress without turning to food. Here are some ideas:

- Take a walk.
- Listen to music.
- Call a friend.

- Practice breathing techniques or yoga.
- Take a warm bath.
- Work on a hobby.
- Meditate.
- Play with your pet.
- Hug someone.
- Don't be afraid to ask for help if things don't improve.

Practice Your ABCs Every Day

A — Adequate Activity
B — Breakfast every morning
C — Calcium
D — Drink plenty of water
E — Eat regular meals
F — Fiber, fruits and vegetables

Have a Positive Attitude

- Believe in yourself.
- Like yourself for who you are now.
- Don't spend time worrying about unimportant things.
- Make time for fun too.
- Don't give up if things don't progress as fast as you would like them to.

Get Support

- Involve your family to the extent that you are able and feel comfortable.
- Surround yourself with supportive friends who have your best interests at heart.

Appendix B: Medical Conditions Causing or Associated with Obesity

More details on the following conditions can be found in chapter 2.

Genetic Syndromes

Prader-Willi syndrome   Down syndrome
Bardet-Biedl syndrome   Cohen syndrome
Alstrom syndrome

Single Gene Mutations/Defects

Mutation in the leptin receptor gene
Mutation in the melanocortin 4 receptor gene (a gene that seems to play
    a role in controlling eating behavior)

Hormonal Problems

Hypothyroidism
Cushing syndrome
Conditions involving the hypothalamus
Hyperinsulinemia (elevated insulin levels)

Other Medical Conditions

- Polycystic ovary syndrome.
- Certain medications such as steroids and medications used to treat depression and mood disorders can contribute to weight gain.

Appendix C:
Resources

Academy for Eating Disorders
6728 Old McLean Village Drive
McLean VA 22101
(703) 556-9222
www.acadeatdis.org

American Academy of Pediatrics
141 Northwest Point Boulevard
Elk Grove Village IL 60009-0927
www.aap.org

American Dietetic Association
120 South Riverside Plaza, Suite
  2000
Chicago IL 60606-6995
(800) 877-1600
Nutrition information line
(800) 366-1655
www.eatright.org

American Obesity Association
1250 24th Street N.W., Suite 300
Washington D.C. 20037
(202) 776-7711
www.obesity.org

Anorexia Nervosa and Related
  Eating Disorders (ANRED)
(541) 344-1144
www.anred.com

Centers for Disease Control and
  Prevention
1600 Clifton Road
Atlanta GA 30333
(800) 311-3435
www.cdc.gov

Gurze Books
www.bulimia.com

National Association of Anorexia
  Nervosa and Associated Disorders (ANAD)
P.O. Box 7
Highland Park IL 60035
(847) 831-3438
www.anad.org

National Eating Disorders Association
603 Stewart Street, Suite 803
Seattle WA 98101
(206) 382-3587
Eating disorders information and referral help-line:
(800) 931-2237
www.nationaleatingdisorders.org

National Institute of Child Health and Human Development
31 Center Drive
Bethesda MD 20892-2425
(301) 496-5133
www.nichd.nih.gov/

National Institute of Diabetes and Digestive and Kidney Disorders
31 Center Drive
Bethesda MD 20892-2560
www.niddk.nih.gov

National Institutes of Health
Bethesda MD
www.nih.gov

North American Association for the Study of Obesity
8630 Fenton Street, Suite 918
Silver Spring MD 20910
(301) 563-6526
www.naaso.org

Suburban Center for Eating Disorders and Adolescent Obesity
6410 Rockledge Drive, Suite 410
Bethesda MD 20817
(301) 530-0676
www.suburbanhospital.org

Glossary

Aerobic activity— an activity that involves sustained exercise, requiring the use of oxygen, e.g. running, biking, rowing, dancing.

Anorexia nervosa— an eating disorder in which the individual is significantly underweight due to restriction of calorie intake, has a fear of gaining weight, and has a disturbance in body image. Girls who have begun menstruating, stop, because a minimum amount of fat is needed for hormone function.

Autosomal recessive— a type of genetic inheritance requiring both parents (of the affected individual) to be carriers of the gene.

Basal metabolic rate (BMR)— the rate at which energy is used by a person or organism at rest.

Basal metabolism— the amount of energy required by an organism to perform only basic vital functions (such as breathing) at rest.

Behavior modification— the use of learning techniques to modify behaviors, i.e. to change undesirable behavior to more desirable behavior.

Binge eating/Bingeing— eating large amounts of food in a limited period of time with a feeling of loss of control over the eating behavior.

Binge-eating disorder— an eating disorder characterized by recurrent episodes of binge eating over a prolonged period of time (at least six months).

Body-mass index— a weight-for-height measure that is an indication of body fat status.

Bulimia nervosa— an eating disorder in which the individual develops regular episodes of binge eating, as well as some compensatory mechanism to get rid of the extra calories. This could take the form of vomiting, use of pills, dieting or excessive exercising.

Calorie— the amount of energy required to raise the temperature of 1 gram of water by 1 degree centigrade at 1 atmosphere pressure. (The correct term to use is really "kilocalorie," but we use the term calorie for short.)

Carbohydrates— a group of organic compounds that provide a major source of energy in the diet, and include sugars, starches and cellulose.

Cushing syndrome— a metabolic syndrome caused by an excess of glucocorticoids (cortisol) in the body.

Diabetes mellitus— a metabolic disorder caused by too little production of insulin by the pancreas, or insulin resistance, and characterized by high blood glucose levels.

Dietitian— someone who specializes in the study of nutrition and the role nutrition plays in health.

Exercise physiologist— a clinical exercise physiologist specializes in the use of physical activity and the development of exercise programs to achieve health and functional benefits, including muscular and cardiovascular conditioning.

FDA— the FDA (Food and Drug Administration) is a U.S. federal agency responsible for regulating the release of new foods and health-related products.

Fad diet— a diet that is unusual, extreme, or "popular" and is not based on sound scientific evidence.

Fiber—"roughage" or indigestible plant matter.

Food journal/food diary— any book which is used to record one's intake of food and drink.

Gastric bypass surgery— surgery sometimes used to treat morbid (severe) obesity.

Gene— a hereditary unit located on a chromosome, and capable of determining a specific characteristic in an organism.

Genotype— the genetic "make-up" of an individual.

Hirsutism— the presence of excessive hair on the face or body.

Hypercholesterolemia— a condition in which blood cholesterol is abnormally high.

Hypertension—high blood pressure.

Hypothyroidism—underactivity of the thyroid gland, which secretes thyroid hormones. Thyroid hormones help regulate metabolism, and insufficient production of thyroid hormones can lead to tiredness, cold intolerance, weight gain and hair loss.

Insulin—a hormone secreted by the pancreas, which plays a role in blood glucose regulation.

Insulin resistance—a condition in which there is less-effective functioning of insulin, leading to poor regulation of blood glucose. Insulin resistance can be associated with obesity.

Metabolism—the processes occurring within an organism, that are necessary to maintain life.

Obese—very overweight, due to excessive body fat.

Osteopenia—a condition in which there is decreased bone density ("thinning of the bones"), but not to the point of having osteoporosis.

Osteoporosis—a condition in which there is extreme loss of bone density, and an increased risk of bone fracture.

Pedometer—an instrument used to record the number of steps taken within a period of time.

Phenylketonuria (PKU)—a genetic disorder in which a person lacks the enzyme needed to convert phenylalanine to tyrosine. If untreated, this can lead to brain damage.

Polycystic ovary syndrome—a disease of the ovaries associated with clinical symptoms such as obesity, irregular menstruation and hirsutism.

Protein—components of all living cells, and essential in the diet for growth and repair of tissue; found in foods such as meat, fish, legumes, milk and eggs.

Purging—a means of ridding the body of extra calories (in the case of bulimia) by self-induced vomiting or the use of pills such as diuretics or laxatives.

Resistance training—strength training, or use of resistance methods such as free weights, machines or body weight to strengthen muscles.

Glossary

Resting heart rate— heart rate taken at complete rest, preferably before rising in the morning.

Satiety (satiation)—feeling of fullness or having one's hunger satisfied.

Saturated fat—fat made up of chains of saturated fatty acids, an excess of which can raise blood cholesterol levels and put one at increased risk for heart disease.

Sedentary activity— an activity that involves sitting and is not active; an example is watching television.

Shin splints— an overuse injury of the lower leg.

Strength training— see resistance training.

Unsaturated fat—fat made up of chains of unsaturated fatty acids.

Vegan diet— a diet excluding all animal products including milk and eggs.

Vegetarian diet— a diet consisting of mostly vegetables, fruits, grains, nuts and seeds, with or without eggs and dairy products.

Vitamin— a substance essential in very small amounts for normal growth and activity of the body, and obtained naturally from plant and animal foods.

Yo-yo dieting— weight cycling, or a repeated pattern of losing and then regaining body weight.

Bibliography

Books

Allison, Kelly C., Albert J. Stunkard, and Sara L. Thier. *Overcoming Night Eating Syndrome*. Oakland, CA: New Harbinger Publications, 2004.

American Academy of Pediatrics. *Pediatric Nutrition Handbook*. 5th ed. Edited by Ronald E. Kleinman, M.D. Elk Grove Village, IL: American Academy of Pediatrics, 2004.

Andersen, Arnold, Leigh Cohn, and Thomas Holbrook. *Making Weight: Men's Conflicts with Food, Weight, Shape and Appearance*. Carlsbad, CA: Gurze, 2000.

Behrman, Richard E., Robert Kliegman, and Hal Jenson. *Nelson Textbook of Pediatrics*. 17th ed. Philadelphia: Saunders, 2004.

Berg, Frances. *Underage & Overweight: America's Childhood Obesity Crisis — What Every Family Needs to Know*. New York: Hatherleigh Press, 2004.

Borushek, Allan. *The Doctor's Pocket Calorie Fat & Carbohydrate Counter*. Costa Mesa, CA: Family Health Publications, 2004.

Brownell, Kelly D., and Katherine Battle Horgen. *Food Fight*. New York: McGraw Hill/Contemporary Books, 2004.

Davis, Brangien. *What's Real, What's Ideal: Overcoming a Negative Body Image*. Center City, MN: Hazelden, 1999.

Diagnostic and Statistical Manual of Mental Disorders. 4th ed., text revision. Washington, DC: American Psychiatric Association, 2000.

Duyff, Roberta Larson. *The American Dietetic Association's Complete Food and Nutrition Guide*. 2d ed. New York: John Wiley & Sons, 2002.

Fairburn, Christopher G. *Overcoming Binge Eating*. New York: Guilford Press, 1995.

_____, and Kelly D. Brownell. *Eating Disorders and Obesity: A Comprehensive Handbook*. 2d ed. New York: Guilford Press, 2002.

Heller, Tania. *Eating Disorders: A Handbook for Teens, Families and Teachers*. Jefferson, NC: McFarland, 2003.

Litt, A. *Fuel for Young Athletes: Essential Foods and Fluids for Future Champions*. Champaign, IL: Human Kinetics, 2004.

Bibliography

Mitchell, James E. *The Outpatient Treatment of Eating Disorders: A Guide for Therapists, Dieticians and Physicians.* Minneapolis: University of Minnesota Press, 2001.

Ravage, Barbara. *K.I.S.S. Guide to Weight Loss.* New York,: Dorling Kindersley, 2001.

Richardson, B. L., and E. Rehr. *101 Ways to Help Your Daughter Love Her Body.* New York: HarperCollins, 2001.

Satter, Ellyn. *How to Get Your Kid to Eat... But Not Too Much.* Boulder, CO: Bull Publishing Co., 1987.

Sears, William, and Martha Sears. *The Family Nutrition Book.* New York: Little, Brown, 1999.

Sharma, Robin S. *The Monk Who Sold His Ferrari: A Fable About Fulfilling Your Dreams and Reaching Your Destiny.* New York: HarperCollins, 1997.

Siegel, Michele, Judith Brisman, and Margot Weinshel. *Surviving an Eating Disorder: Strategies for Family and Friends.* New York: HarperPerennial, 1997.

Sothern, Melinda S., T. Kristian von Almen, and Heidi Schumacher. *Trim Kids.* New York: Quill/HarperResource, 2001.

Wadden, Thomas, and Albert Stunkard. *Handbook of Obesity Treatment.* New York: Guilford Press, 2002.

Articles

Academy for Eating Disorders. "Parental Influences on Eating Behavior in Obese and Nonobese Preadolescents." *International Journal of Eating Disorders.* December 2001, 30 (4).

Ackard DM, Neumark-Sztainer D, Story M, Perry C. "Overeating among Adolescents: Prevalence and Associations with Weight-Related Characteristics and Psychological Health." *Pediatrics.* January 2003, 111 (1): 67–74.

American Academy of Pediatrics. Committee on Adolescence. "Policy Statement: Identifying and Treating Eating Disorders." *Pediatrics.* January 2003, 111 (1): 204–211.

American Academy of Pediatrics. Committee on Nutrition. "Prevention of Pediatric Overweight and Obesity." *Pediatrics.* August 2003, 112 (2): 424–430.

American Academy of Pediatrics. Committee on Nutrition. "Soft Drinks Replacing Healthier Alternatives in American Diet." *AAP News.* January 2002, 20 (1): 36

American Academy of Pediatrics. Committee on Nutrition. "The Use and Misuse of Fruit Juice in Pediatrics." *Pediatrics.* May 2001, 107 (5): 1210–1213.

Bibliography

American Academy of Pediatrics. Committee on Public Education. "Children, Adolescents, and Television." *Pediatrics.* February 2001, 107 (2): 423–426.

American Academy of Pediatrics. Committee on School Health. "Policy Statement: Soft Drinks in Schools." *Pediatrics.* January 2004, 113(1): 152–154.

American Academy of Pediatrics. Committee on Sports Medicine and Fitness and Committee on School Health. "Organized Sports for Children and Preadolescents." *Pediatrics.* June 2001, 107 (6): 1459–1462.

American Academy of Pediatrics. Committee on Sports Medicine and Fitness and Committee on School Health. "Physical Fitness and Activity in Schools." *Pediatrics.* May 2000, 105 (5): 1156–1157.

American Academy of Pediatrics. Committee on Sports Medicine and Fitness. "Strength Training by Children and Adolescents." *Pediatrics.* June 2001, 107 (6): 1470–1472.

Amisola RVB, Jacobson MS. "Physical Activity, Exercise, and Sedentary Activity: Relationship to the Causes and Treatment of Obesity. *Adolescent Medicine.* February 2003, 14 (1).

Barry DT, Grilo CM, Masheb RM. "Gender Differences in Patients with Binge Eating Disorder." *International Journal of Eating Disorders.* January 2002, 31 (1).

Bonow RO, Gheorghiade M. "The Diabetes Epidemic: A National and Global Crisis." *American Journal of Medicine.* March 2004, 116 (5), Suppl. 1.

Bowman SA, Gortmaker SL, Ebbeling CB, Pereira MA, Ludwig DS. "Effects of Fast-Food Consumption on Energy Intake and Diet Quality Among Children in a National Household Survey." *Pediatrics.* January 2004, 113 (1): 112–118.

Branson R, Potoczna N, Kral JG, Lentes KU, Hoehe MR, Horber FF. "Binge Eating as a Major Phenotype of Melanocortin 4 Receptor Gene Mutations." *New England Journal of Medicine.* March 2003, 348 (12).

Brown WM, Sibille K, Phelps L, McFarlane KJ. "Obesity in Children and Adolescents." (Review Article) *Clinics in Family Practice.* September 2002, 4 (3).

Brownell, K. D. "Fast Food and Obesity in Children." *Pediatrics.* January 2004, 113 (1): 132 (part 1 of 2).

Butler MG, Bittel DC, Kibiryeva N, Talebizadeh Z, Thompson T. "Behavioral Differences among Subjects with Prader-Willi Syndrome and Type I or Type II Deletion and Maternal Disomy." *Pediatrics.* March 2004, 113 (3): 565–573.

Castellani W, Ianni L, Ricca V, Mannucci E, and Rotella CM. "Adherence to Structured and Physical Exercise in Overweight and Obese Subjects: A Review of Psychological Models." *Eating and Weight Disorders.* March 2003, 8 (1): 1–11.

Bibliography

Centers for Disease Control and Prevention. "Update: Prevalence of Overweight among Children, Adolescents, and Adults: United States, 1988–1994." *MMWR*. March 1997, 46 (9): 198–202.

Certain LK, Kahn RS. "Prevalence, Correlates, and Trajectory of Television Viewing Among Infants and Toddlers." *Pediatrics*. April 2002, 109 (4): 634–642.

Crawford, PB, Story M, Wang MC, Ritchie LD and Sabry ZI. "Childhood and Adolescent Obesity: Ethnic Issues in the Epidemiology of Childhood Obesity." *Pediatric Clinics of North America*. August 2001, 48 (4).

Donohoue PA. "Obesity." Chapter 43 in Behrman et al., *Nelson Textbook of Pediatrics*. Philadelphia: Saunders, 2004.

Dorian L, Garfinkel PE. "Culture and Body Image in Western Society." *Eating and Weight Disorders: Studies on Anorexia, Bulimia and Obesity*. March 2002, 7 (1).

Faith MS, Berman N, et al. "Effects of Contingent Television on Physical Activity and Television Viewing in Obese Children." *Pediatrics*. May 2001, 107 (5).

Faith MS, Pietrobelli A, Nunez C, Heo M, Heymsfield SB, Allison DB. "Evidence for Independent Genetic Influences on Fat Mass and Body Mass Index in a Pediatric Twin Sample." *Pediatrics*. July 1999, 104 (1): 61–67.

Foreyt JP and Poston WSC. "Consensus View on the Role of Dietary Fat and Obesity." *American Journal of Medicine*. December 2002, 113 (Suppl. 9B).

Freedman DS, Khan LK, Dietz WH, Srinivasan SR, Berenson GS. "Relationship of Childhood Obesity to Coronary Heart Disease Risk Factors in Adulthood: The Bogalusa Heart Study." *Pediatrics*. September 2001, 108 (3).

Hyder ML, O'Byrne KK, Poston WSC, Foreyt JP. "Behavior Modification in the Treatment of Obesity." *Clinics in Family Practice*. June 2002, 4 (2)

Janz KF, Burns TL, Torner JC, Levy SM, Paulos R, Willing MC, Warren JJ. "Physical Activity and Bone Measures in Young Children: The Iowa Bone Development Study." *Pediatrics*. June 2001, 107 (6): 1387–1393.

Jay MS. "Childhood Obesity Is Not PHAT!" *Journal of Pediatrics*. April 2004, 144 (4).

Jonides L, Buschbacher V, Barlow SE. "Management of Child and Adolescent Obesity: Psychological, Emotional, and Behavioral Assessment." *Pediatrics*. July 2002, 110 (1): 215–221.

Kaplowitz PB, Slora EJ, Wasserman RC, et al. "Earlier Onset of Puberty in Girls: Relation to Increased Body Mass Index and Race." *Pediatrics*. August 2001, 108 (2): 347–353.

Kazaks A, Stern JS. "Obesity: Food Intake." *Primary Care; Clinics in Office Practice*. June 2003, 30 (2).

Kimm SYS, Obarzanek E. "Childhood Obesity: A New Pandemic of the New Millennium." *Pediatrics*. November 2002, 110 (5): 1003–1007.

Bibliography

Levine MD, Ringham RM, Kalarchian MA, Wisniewski L, Marcus MD. "Is Family-Based Behavioral Weight Control Appropriate for Severe Pediatric Obesity?" *International Journal of Eating Disorders.* November 2001, 30 (3): 318–328.

Maynard LM, Wisemandle W, Roche AF, Chumlea WC, Guo SS, Siervogel RM. "Childhood Body Composition in Relation to Body Mass Index." *Pediatrics.* February 2001, 107 (2): 344–350.

McCaffree J. "Childhood Eating Patterns: The Roles Parents Play." *Journal of the American Dietetic Association.* December 2003, 103 (12): 1587.

Moilanen C. "Vegan Diets in Infants, Children, and Adolescents." *Pediatrics in Review.* May 2004, 25 (5).

Nichter M. "Listening to Girls Talk About Their Bodies." *Reclaiming Children and Youth.* Fall 2000, 9 (13): 182.

O'Brien P, Dixon JB. "The Extent of the Problem of Obesity." *American Journal of Surgery.* December 2002, 184 (6B).

Ogden CL, Troiano RP, Briefel RR, et al. "Prevalence of Overweight Among Preschool Children in the United States, 1971–1994." *Pediatrics.* April 1997, 99 (4).

Pratt HD, Patel DR, Greydanus DE. "Behavioral Aspects of Children's Sports." *Pediatric Clinics of North America.* August 2003, 50 (4).

Rowell HA, Evans BJ, Quarry-Horn JL, Kerrigan JR. "Adolescent Endocrinology: Type 2 Diabetes Mellitus in Adolescents." *Adolescent Medicine.* February 2002, 13 (1).

Salbe AD, Weyer C, Lindsay RS, Ravussin E, Tataranni PA. "Assessing Risk Factors for Obesity between Childhood and Adolescence: I. Birth Weight, Childhood Adiposity, Parental Obesity, Insulin, and Leptin." *Pediatrics.* August 2002, 110 (2) 299–306.

_____, _____, Harper I, Lindsay RS, Ravussin E, Tataranni PA. "Assessing Risk Factors for Obesity between Childhood and Adolescence: II. Energy Metabolism and Physical Activity." *Pediatrics.* August 2002, 110 (2): 307–314.

Sorbara M, Geliebter A. "Body Image Disturbance in Obese Outpatients before and after Weight Loss in Relation to Race, Gender, Binge Eating, and Age of Onset of Obesity." *International Journal of Eating Disorder.* May 2002, 31 (4): 416–423.

Sorof JM, Lai D, Turner J, Poffenbarger T, Portman RJ. "Overweight, Ethnicity, and the Prevalence of Hypertension in School-Aged Children." Pediatrics. March 2004, 113 (3): 475–482.

Sothern MS. "Childhood and Adolescent Obesity. Exercise as a Modality in the Treatment of Childhood Obesity." *Pediatric Clinics of North America.* August 2001, 48 (4).

Steinberger J, et al. "Adiposity in Childhood Predicts Obesity and Insulin

Bibliography

Resistance in Young Adulthood." *Journal of Pediatrics.* April 2001, 138 (4): 469–473.

Tomeo CA, Field AE, Berkey CS, Colditz GA, Frazier AL. "Weight Concerns, Weight Control Behaviors, and Smoking Initiation." *Pediatrics.* October 1999, 104 (4): 918–924.

Trowbridge FL, Sofka D, Holt K, Barlow SE. "Management of Child and Adolescent Obesity: Study Design and Practitioner Characteristics." *Pediatrics.* July 2002, 110 (1): 205–209.

Weaver CM, Boushey CJ. "Milk — Good for Bones, Good for Reducing Childhood Obesity?" *Journal of the American Dietetic Association.* December 2003,103 (12): 1598–1599.

White MA, Kohlmaier JR, Varnado-Sullivan P, Williamson DA. "Racial/ Ethnic Differences in Weight Concerns: Protective and Risk Factors for the Development of Eating Disorders and Obesity Among Adolescent Females." *Eating and Weight Disorders. Studies on Anorexia, Bulimia and Obesity.* March 2003, 8 (1): 20–25.

Wyatt HR. "The prevalence of obesity." *Primary Care; Clinics in Office Practice.* June 2003, 30 (2).

Zametkin AJ, Zoon CZ, Klein HW, Munson S. "Psychiatric Aspects of Child and Adolescent Obesity: A Review of the Past 10 Years." *Journal of the American Academy of Child and Adolescent Psychiatry.* February 2004, 43 (2).

Index

Index

insulin 37; resistance 20, 37
insurance 53
iron deficiency 1, 71

joints 39

lanugo hair 120
leptin 20, 164
low-density lipoprotein 38, 68

media 46, 134, 149
melanocortin 4 receptor gene 20, 164
Meridia 100
metabolic syndrome 37
metabolism 4, 75
Metformin 61
Middle East 10
minerals 71
mono-unsaturated fats 67
mortality 39

Native American 10
neuropeptide Y 20
night eating syndrome 22

obesity: assessment 51–53; causes 11–26; complications 36–43; definition and prevalence 7–10; guide for parents 123–146; maintaining a healthy lifestyle 101–113; prevention 147–149; treatment 54–100
organized sports 82
Orlistat 99
osteopenia 119
osteoporosis 119, 155

pedometer 84
personal trainers 84
phenylketonuria 154
physical activity 79–88, 109, 133
physical education 16–17
Pilates 82
polycystic ovary syndrome 20, 39, 165
poly-unsaturated fats 67
portions 14, 64–66
poverty 17
Prader-Willi syndrome 19, 164

prejudice 40
protein 69
psychotherapy 98–99
puberty 47

questionnaire 23

safety 16
saturated fats 67
school lunches 146
self-esteem 4, 40, 44–50, 111–112, 135–136
serving size 66
set-backs 111
shopping list 143–144
Sibutramine 99–100
sleep 110–111
sleep apnea 38
Slim-Fast 33
smoking 10, 42
society 22, 149
South Africa 10
stroke 37
Stunkard, Albert 22

teasing 41, 140
television 16–17, 85, 140
thrifty genes 21
Time magazine 18
trans fats 67
traveling 105–107
triglycerides 37

vegan 72
vegetarian 72
vitamins 70

water 71–72
weight-loss camps 136–137
Weight Watchers 33

Xenical 99

yoga 81–82, 163
yo-yo dieting 16, 140, 159

zinc 71